The Answer to AIDS –

from **St. Louis...**

Deborah Latchison

Note for Librarians: A cataloguing record for this book is available from Library and Archives Canada at www.collectionscanada.ca/amicus/index-e.html
ISBN 1-4120-8836-4

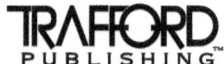

PUBLISHING™

Offices in Canada, USA, Ireland and UK

Book sales for North America and international:
Trafford Publishing, 6E–2333 Government St.,
Victoria, BC V8T 4P4 CANADA
phone 250 383 6864 (toll-free 1 888 232 4444)
fax 250 383 6804; email to orders@trafford.com
Book sales in Europe:
Trafford Publishing (UK) Limited, 9 Park End Street, 2nd Floor
Oxford, UK OX1 1HH UNITED KINGDOM
phone +44 (0)1865 722 113 (local rate 0845 230 9601)
facsimile +44 (0)1865 722 868; info.uk@trafford.com
Order online at:
trafford.com/06-0592
10 9 8 7 6 5 4 3 2

Table of Contents

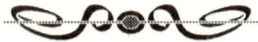

This Book is Dedicated to the
Memory of Esther Ruth...

When I began gathering data for this book two years ago my beautiful, precocious niece, Esther Ruth, wanted to contribute. Mind you, she was aware that only members of the clergy had been asked for input – but nine year old Esther had something she wanted to say and was not about to be deterred or intimidated by particulars. I stopped production of this book to include what she wrote:

"Solution…"

"AIDS has been spreading for quite some time. Women, if I was you I would go every month and get my husband and self a blood test. If your husband doesn't want to take the test, women, he probably has something to hide. Men, if you want your wife, girlfriend or fiance to stick around, don't fool around – or there might be no women left."

By:
Esther Ruth Nichols
9 years old

Esther attended school on May 3, 2006. But later on that day, my brilliant niece was tragically killed in a car accident while riding with her mother and my sister, Ruth. They were hit by a drunk driver.

I miss you, Esther Ruth…

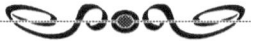

To my children, Nicole Carmelle and Charles Paul, Jr.

To my Sisters and Brothers

Betty, Andrew, Ruth, Mark, Martha & Samson

"Keep on Believing"…

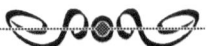

~ Acknowledgments ~

To each pastor, bishop, minister or personal friend who contributed towards the fruition of this project, you have my deepest gratitude: Pastor Charles Roach, Minister Samson N. Latchison (Springfield), Archbishop Michael A. West, Sr., Bishop George White, Jr., Bishop Dr. Wyatt I. Greenlee, Reverend Steve Daniels, Jr. (Minnesota), Reverend Larry Rice for allowing me to talk about "The Conspiracy of Silence" on his TV program, Evangelist Ruth Latchison Nichols, Reverend Isaac C. McCullough, Reverend Earl E. Nance, Jr., Reverend Sammie E. Jones for allowing me to address the St. Louis Clergy Coalition regarding AIDS in April 2004, Sheila Grigsby, Pastor Lamarr Goldman, Reverend Carl S. Smith, Sr., Dr. Ralph Petty, Pastor Doug Batchelor (amazingfacts.org), Elder Andrew Latchison, Jr., Pastor Patricia Rattler, Minister Annette Fields, Mr. John I. Payne (Texas), Ms. Bonita Scott. And thank you, Phil, for your encouragement to write this book…

To Mrs. Jean Gore (you are *such* a special lady…)

To a very special group of people, the Jehovah's Witnesses, who watch the world as it fulfills Bible prophesy. I am fascinated by their comprehension of *everything*! Special thanks to Ray Miller and Tanya Robinson for the Watchtower Bible & Tract Society information, and all the wonderful book and Bible studies.

"There is a higher self in man and woman and there is a lower self... We can act like the beasts of the field and we can act like God. The difference between acting like God and reflecting God or acting like the lower animals is how well we obey Allah (God). In obedience to Allah, there is life; in rejection and rebellion to Allah, there is the death of the power that Allah has given us to reflect Him"...

The Honorable Minister Louis Farrakhan

Introduction

Just when we began to live as if the "death-by-disease" angel had died itself, that the scourge of plague had been eradicated forever and that anyone who contracted HIV/AIDS after 1990 was invincible, we have been hit by ever more devastating news: there are more diseases now than ever before and HIV/AIDS infections are *out of control*. In spite of the many technological, medicinal and political advancements made in the last century, man yet is incapable to eradicate, or even *control*, disease.

Yes, disease has plagued mankind unceasingly. The Black Death of the 14th century killed about 20 million people in three years, and it was not known until years later that the disease was caused by rats. The Spanish influenza, which seemingly came from *nowhere* during the early 20th century, killed 20-40 million people worldwide in *one year*. Malaria, smallpox, polio...

However, AIDS is the *only* disease known to mankind – with its devastating ability to destroy life – that can be directly attributed to some form of human activity. In other words, the disease *could* have been prevented and can even now be eradicated by the cessation of the specific human activity providing impetus. After 25 years, however, the United Nations issued the warning in April 2005 that the HIV/AIDS dilemma – though already pandemic – is accelerating. In a November 2006 report, the World Health Organization and UNAIDS projected that by 2010 the life expectancy in many affected countries would drop below 40 years of age. They also project that by 2025 over 200 million worldwide will have died because of HIV/AIDS infections.

For the past two years, since April 2004, my mind has been unwaveringly set on bringing awareness of HIV/AIDS to my community, my city: St. Louis – and it has been 'a long row to hoe,' as the old people used to say. This historical town in which I was born and bred is also home to some of the greatest actors, athletes, scholars, some of the greatest artists, singers and musicians the world has known. Rich in culture, architectural splendor, world-renown hospitals and universities, fantastic sports teams, prominent politicians and sheer natural beauty, St. Louis is an alluring city -- with the magnificent, towering *Gateway Arch* as the ultimate beacon.

But behind the lighted splendor, glitz and glamour there exists a conspiracy of silence regarding AIDS in this community, which is due mainly to St. Louis' deeply planted roots in the ground of rigid conservatism – a city where even the polarities have polarities – cultural, societal, economic, political, religious and educational. Hence, no one wants to talk about 'it'. The issue causes people to become *uncomfortable*, to fidget and squirm – as if 'it' were a deep, dark secret that is never to be mentioned, nor revealed. Most act as if the disease will just disappear, or improve, simply by ignoring it. AIDS is no longer a novelty issue, so attitudes here are apathetic. Indifference prevails even though current figures are closer to those of 1995 than in the last few years. And *that* just grinds my beans...

I was asked once what qualified me to write this book. I am not a doctor, or even a healthcare professional. I have not accumulated any course credits in studying this disease and do not work at any of the local agencies. Perhaps the only qualification I possess is that I *choose* to talk about this subject in an effort to bring consciousness regarding the gravity of this disease -- especially for the sake of young people -- because *I care*. Plus, from the *angst* involved in writing this book, I've watched the small trashcan in my bathroom fill up with my once shoulder-length hair and dime-sized boils break out over my body. Aw, it's *on* now, baby...

This book was written to point out the danger of HIV/AIDS' unperceived threat in America and shed light on the fact that AIDS is primarily a *heterosexual* disease here – and nearly totally black. This book will reveal the unfortunate reality of the causes of the disease's propagation in this country due to arrogance, ignorance, denial – and the *horrendous* absence of sexual integrity, sexual responsibility and sexual discipline. We have been mistaken in assuming that our behaviors would not demand reprisal.

My desire from the start in writing this book is that it not be considered 'religious' in *any* form -- but rather a *spiritual*, informational resource that will be referred to as a comprehensive aid in healing humans' physical, sexual and Godly relationships. I am especially hopeful that communication will be encouraged between parents and children, between the church, parents and children, and to engage young people in right thinking on their views regarding sex, as opposed to the conflicting misinformation they are exposed to on a constant basis by various forms. Optimistically, what is written within these pages will define the human experience in its truest, most spiritual context, define the self-destructive, base consequences of exploitative, promiscuous behaviors and explain our purpose in connection to a loving God…

In final preparation to send this book to press, it troubled me that I really hadn't enough information to explain in greater detail the origin of AIDS. It *is* known, however, that HIV/AIDS infection is *totally dependent upon human participation* to exist and propagate. In other words, AIDS starts *and* stops with us. Currently, there are only two activities by which one can contract the disease: having sex with an infected person, or drug use. Not only *intravenous* drug use (using 'dirty' needles) but a person with a monkey on his back is apt to sell his body to acquire money for more drugs.

That is when the focus of my attention was suddenly shifted to a much larger screen, and my thought process transferred from the disease itself to issues that I perceived *actually birthed* the disease. It went from being about only HIV/AIDS statistics to the various human deficiencies, a.k.a. '**A**cquired **I**mmune **D**eficiencie**S**', or **AIDS** of the four components that comprise our existence: family, church, politics and society. I was nearly blown away! You see, it doesn't matter whether we find a cure for AIDS *today* because unless something changes, *other* diseases will be bred even more virulent than AIDS has been. What is really needed is a change in *people*, in *us*. When *we* change, STDs will be abated, family, church, politics and society will all be fixed – because *people* formulate all these factions…

Have you ever applied antiseptic to an open wound? It *hurts,* doesn't it? The *truth* is like antiseptic applied to an open wound – it *burns* – and will even burn any other scratched or wounded area in close proximity. Sometimes we have wounds that we were totally unaware of until antiseptic is applied to *another* area. But antiseptic is necessary towards the prevention of further infection and hastening the *healing* process. It cleanses the wound and removes all impurities and when it *burns*, you know it is working. So it is with *truth*. If anything in this book causes you to 'burn', (1) you clearly have an open wound in that area; (2) you need to seriously analyze the area that hurts for the presence of 'infection' and (3) swab the 'sore' spot with a healthy application of the antiseptic of truth. It will bring you healing, happiness and *freedom* in no time flat…

Just So You Know…

Before proceeding to accomplish the task at hand, it is essential that the proper groundwork be laid, a strong foundation established to support whatever is built upon it. The *tools,* also, of any trade are essential to the accomplishment of the task. To be an attorney one must have access to and be trained to use the tools of that trade. This rule applies whether you're a doctor, engineer or street sweeper. So it is with this assignment – the proper utensils must be selected to suitably address the task at hand.

This book will deal with some extremely weighty issues regarding human nature and will, therefore, require the most precise, heavy-duty equipment that is available. This equipment must be effective, possess the ability to reach to the very core of the problem and conflict, uproot and pluck out even the deepest innate deficiencies. Therefore, I have chosen the Bible as my major reference tool and informational source of truth. The Bible is the most *effective* instrument available to define and remedy the human condition -- a bona fide "User's Manual", if you will.

Who would know more about a piece of art than the artist who created it? Who would know more about a building than the architect who built it? And who would know more about human behavior than the Creator of us all, and the author of the Bible - Jehovah God?

The Bible is dependable, historically and scientifically accurate. Above all, it is the inspired Word of God. The oldest portion of the Bible dates back to the 16th century B.C. This is before the appearance of the Hindu *Rig-Veda* (in about 1300 B.C.), or the Buddhist "Canon of the Three Baskets" (fifth century B.C.), or the Islamic Koran (seventh century C.E.), as well as the Shinto *Nihongi* (720 C.E.).

To interpolate, in believing that the Bible is the inspired Word of God we must believe that it is either *all true*, or that *none* of it is true. In other words, you cannot pick and choose just *portions* of the Bible in which to believe. There are times when we have no trouble believing one part of the Bible as being the inspired Word of God, yet disbelieve other portions that offend us or that we disagree with. It is all written in the *same book.*

Life's deepest and most disturbing questions are answered in the Bible. The late Indian leader Mohandas K. Gandhi reportedly told a British official: "When your country and mine shall get together on the teachings laid down by Christ in this Sermon on the Mount, we shall have solved the problems not only of our countries but those of the whole world."

The Bible is reliable. *"Heaven and earth shall pass away, but my words will not pass away"* (Matthew 24:35). Mighty kingdoms have risen and fallen (Babylon, Medo-Persia, Greece and Rome). Great men have lived and died – but God's word is *alive* and being fulfilled in the earth. *"I am the Lord... new things do I declare: before they spring forth I tell you of them"* (Isaiah 42:8, 9. *"I am God... Declaring the end from the beginning, and from ancient times the things that are not yet done."* (Isaiah 46:9,10).

The wise man, Solomon, once wrote: *"There is nothing new under the sun. Whatever has been will be again" (Ecclesiastes 3:15).* Time has proven him to be correct – for even though mankind is continually developing 'new' technologies it is all *relative.* Fire was considered new to cavemen in ancient times. At one point in human history, the wheel was considered an ingenious invention – and new. No matter what mankind invents, it is only new and unique to a particular moment or period. However, the wise man Solomon also wrote, *"I know that whatever God does shall be forever..."* (Ecclesiastes 3:14). And perhaps the one thing we can agree on and that the Bible states: *'a man that is born of a woman is of but a few days and those days are filled with trouble'* (Job 14:1). Be assured that the information provided in this book is derived from the most reliable source there is – the Word of God...

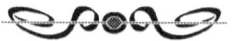

CHAPTER I

THE CRISIS

"The enemy is us…"

Historically, prior to major shifts in social attitudes certain incidents preceded these shifts and, in fact, set the stage for their arrival. In the past, changes in philosophical and psychological thinking have had a worldwide, blanket affect that is not easily understood. However, it *is* understood that attitudes have traditionally been greatly influenced by financial systems, media forms, entertainment and fashion.

The 1960s (or "The Sixties") has come to refer to a complex of inter-related cultural and political events that occurred between 1960 and 1969, mainly in the United States but also in other western countries, particularly France, West Germany and Britain.

The 1960s is the pivotal point in time that stands out as the instant where all systems collided, and exploded into revolution. This era will go down in human witness as a period defined by a spirit of protest, and an inability of people to agree—to agree about almost anything – except the mind-set "anything goes." Its overriding theme was personal freedom and self-fulfillment – 'doing one's own thing.' Never prior to this period had there been such an *effective*, mass rebellion against long-established social, religious and political traditions.

The spirit of protest revealed a *worldwide* breakdown in respect for authority—parental, educational, governmental, and religious. It fostered an atmosphere that frequently led to violence. The wider aspect of the 60's rebellion in the United States reflects a demographic dynamic. The parents of the "Baby-Boom" generation (born between 1945 and 1955) had typically grown up in The Great Depression, served in World War II and started families in the early years of the Cold War. They valued hard work, conventionality and self-discipline. They believed in traditional values, which as they saw it, had made America a great world power and had given them a standard of living their parents in the 1930s did not have.

However, the children of post-war parents, having grown up in affluence and security, did not share these views and valued instead personal freedom above all else. This brought them into conflict with their fathers, university deans, the United States military, President Lyndon Johnson and city police. *Anyone* perceived as an authority figure was to be defied and rebelled against. This violence-laden defiance of authority helped to lay the basic foundation for terrorism. In fact, political analysts have said that modern terrorism began in the 1960s, "clearly the years when a generation born after the last world war declared its *own* war on society."

The beginning of what was happily seen as a new political era with the election of President John F. Kennedy in 1960 was cut unfortunately short, ending in tragedy and disillusionment with Kennedy's assassination in 1963. The United States, in fact, lost *several* impacting leaders of varying social and political agendas to assassins within less than five years: President John F. Kennedy, civil-rights leaders Medgar Evers, Malcolm X and Martin Luther King, Jr., and Senator Robert F. Kennedy.

During the 60's there was also a spirit of *religious* protest, which was not limited to efforts to overhaul conventional religions. The most extreme radicals turned to cultism of various kinds as they lost their faith in political activism. Groups like the Divine Light Mission, Hare Krishna, and the Children of God got their start during the 1960s and grew in enormous popularity. Events such as the mass suicides in Jonestown, orchestrated by cult-leader Jim Jones, represented the remains of 1960s extremism. However, many young Europeans and Americans simply spurned these groups altogether, turning to Asian philosophies.

The 1960s saw the rise of an alternative culture among youth, creating a huge market for rock, blues, jazz and other music forms produced by drug-influenced bands such as: The Beatles, The Grateful Dead, Jefferson Airplane, The Rolling Stones, The Who and The Doors. Also, radical music in the folk tradition pioneered by Bob Dylan was influential. Happy with neither the war nor life, rock stars and pop singers became idols and icons, often mixing inflammatory political statements into their music. Jimi Hendrix, Janis Joplin, Country Joe McDonald, Santana and many others dictated politics, religion, fashion and behavior with their music.

So it was also primarily during the 1960s that a momentous shift in *sexual* attitudes came to fore, spurred on by an array of social events and precipitating the reshaping of America's total structure. The atmosphere of violence, protest and rebellion was motivated by the use of 'psychedelic' drugs, advanced permissive sex and homosexuality. Communal living became popular. This and other lifestyles formerly considered unacceptable were now viewed as being acceptable alternatives.

The sexual revolution of the 60s, in particular, can be credited for significantly altering the traditional landscape of this nation, all of which was to reap a sad fruitage in later years, as we will see on the following pages...

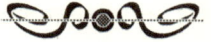

I. The Crisis

Because of the "free love" ethos of the last few decades, which persists to this day, we are experiencing an unprecedented social, medical and personal trouncing by sexual diseases.

The sexual revolution that began in the United States during the 1960s has left two major problems in its wake. The first is the historic increase in non-marital births that have contributed so heavily to the nation's domestic problems including poverty, violence, and inter-generational welfare dependency. The second is the explosion of sexually transmitted diseases (STDs) that now pose an ever-growing hazard to public health. To address these problems, the goal of Federal policy is to emphasize abstinence as the only certain way to avoid both unintended pregnancies and STDs.

Prior to the 60s, there were only two major and known venereal diseases or STDs (sexually transmitted diseases): syphilis and gonorrhea. Today, however, there are more than 40 diseases spread primarily by sexual activity. Together these infectious sexual diseases have created a significant public health challenge in the world. In the United States alone, an estimated 15 million people become infected with one or more STDs *each year*. Because of unbridled sexual freedoms and behaviors of the last few decades, an estimated 65 million people worldwide live with an incurable STD.

Dr. Stanley Falkow stated, "The cartoon character Pogo invented by Walt Kelly once announced to his companions that 'the enemy is us.' I believe that many of what we refer to as emerging diseases is characterized better as 'diseases of human progress.' Thus, many major public health crises of the past two decades have been infectious in origin."

The "miracle drugs" of the past no longer work because bacterial strains of certain primary diseases (e.g., gonorrhea, syphilis, Chlamydia) have mutated and become resistant to conventional medicines. "Antibiotics are rapidly slipping away as a strategy to combat infectious disease," said Dr. Stephen Ostroff, Associate Director of the National Center for Infectious Diseases in Atlanta. Dr. Stuart B. Levy of Tufts University

Medical School said, **"The number of deaths in humans due to drug resistance is going to get worse before it gets better"**.

In 1971, Hepatitis B was found to be sexually transmitted by the CDC (Centers for Disease Control). Then, in 1985 a strain of gonorrhea could no longer be killed by penicillin, the miracle drug developed in the 40s. In 1985, Chlamydia was recognized as the major STD in the United States. In 1989, more cases of congenital syphilis were reported than had been in the 20 years previous.

During the 80s the complexity of STDs increased. Organisms became resistant and the list of STDs grew drastically to include infections due to Chlamydia trachomities, trichomonas vaginalis, genital herpes, bacterial vaginosis, human papilloma virus, enteric pathogens, cytomegalo virus, ectoparasites and hepatitis B.

Now, a most formidable, worldwide killer is on the scene: **AIDS**. After 25 years (first identified in 1981) as the world's most mysterious killer disease of all time, the **AIDS** (Acquired Immuno**D**eficiency Syndrome) virus **has ended more than 25 million lives**. In a May 2006 report stating that the pandemic is accelerating rather than abating, the World Health Organization (WHO) and UNAIDS project that the next 25 years in AIDS may be worse than the last 25 years. These organizations also project that by 2010, **life expectancy in many affected countries will drop below 40 years of age!** (November 2006 *"HIV/AIDS Policy Fact Sheet: Global Overview of the Epidemic,"* issued by The Henry J. Kaiser Family Foundation). As many as **200 million could die from AIDS over the next 20 years**, leaving 25 million orphans behind by 2010.

The facts regarding HIV/AIDS are *horrendous*. No other sexually transmitted disease has proved to be as potent, nor as fatally final as AIDS. On the following pages are listed *alarming* local, national and international statistical data. Please pass this information along to anyone you care for...

NOTE: *Please pay close attention to all items <u>underlined</u> or **bolded**)*

United States – HIV (*Human Immunodeficiency Virus*) Estimate

HIV, the disease that causes AIDS, **is the leading cause of death worldwide, among those 15 through 59 years of age** (November 2006 *"HIV/AIDS Policy Fact Sheet: Global Overview of the Epidemic,"* issued by The Henry J. Kaiser Family Foundation). At the end of **2003**, the Centers for Disease Control and Prevention (CDC) estimated **1,039,000 to 1,185,000** persons in the United States were living with HIV or AIDS, with **24-27%** **undiagnosed and unaware** of their HIV infection. A recent TV commercial further clarified this stat: **1 in 4 Americans is HIV/AIDS positive** – but are not aware of it (Trojan condom commercial, April 2006).

Worldwide, most people who are HIV/AIDS infected are unaware of their infection (November 2006 *"HIV/AIDS Policy Fact Sheet: Global Overview of the Epidemic,"* issued by The Henry J. Kaiser Family Foundation).

AIDS (*Acquired ImmunoDeficiency Syndrome*) Cases

Of the more than one million people estimated to be living with HIV/AIDS in the United States, approximately 42% are estimated to have AIDS, 34% to be HIV positive but not yet progressed to AIDS, and the remainder undiagnosed (Glynn, K., Rhodes, P. *"Estimate HIV Prevalence in the United States at the End of 2003"*, June 2005).

Specific United States HIV/AIDS Statistics

- *AIDS cases have been reported in all 50 states the District of Columbia and all United States territories, with these states reporting the highest cumulative number of cases: New York, California, Florida, Texas, New Jersey, Illinois, Pennsylvania, Puerto Rico, Georgia and Maryland*
- ***40,000 new HIV infections*** *occur each year in America, and have not decreased in the last decade. However, recent analyses suggest a potential rise in infections among some populations (See "Impact of HIV/AIDS on Youth Population" below). 42,000 new infections occurred in 2005.*
- ***Over 1 million*** *of this nation's residents are currently living with HIV*

Cumulatively (from 1981 through the end of 2004), an estimated **529,113 deaths** among people with AIDS in America had occurred, including **16,000 in 2004**. Also, more than **940,000 AIDS cases had been diagnosed, including 42,514 in 2004 alone** *(CDC – Division of HIV/AIDS Prevention – Basic Statistics)*.

An estimated 42% to 59% of people living with HIV/AIDS are not in regular HIV care and a recent analysis found that only 55% of people with HIV/AIDS for whom ARV (Antiretroviral Therapy) would likely be recommended were receiving it in 2003 (Teshale, E. et al., *12th Conference on Retroviruses and Opportunistic Infections*, February 2002).

Global Overview of the HIV/AIDS Pandemic

As of January 2006, the Joint United Nations Programme on HIV/AIDS (UNAIDS) and the World Health Organization (WHO) estimate that **AIDS has killed more than 25 million people** since it was first recognized on June 5, 1981. Despite recent, improved access to antiretroviral treatment and care in many regions of the world, **the AIDS epidemic claimed an estimated 2.8 million (between 2.4 and 3.3 million) lives in 2005** of which **more than half a million (570,000) were children**.

Globally, between 33.4 and 46 million people currently live with HIV. In 2005, between 3.4 and 6.2 million people were newly infected. Also in 2005, between 2.4 and 3.3 million people with AIDS died, an increase from 2003 and the highest number since 1981.

Again, **HIV is the leading cause of death worldwide among 15 to 59 year olds**. The Sub-Saharan African region accounts for two-thirds of people living with HIV/AIDS and almost three quarters of HIV-related deaths. In May 2006, the World Health Organization issued a report to ABC News wherein researchers project that by 2025, **100 million in Africa may die from HIV/AIDS** (UNAIDS "Overview of the global AIDS epidemic", *2006 Report on the global AIDS epidemic*).

Russia, India and China are considered "next wave" countries, where large numbers of people are infected with HIV. The Russian Federation has the largest number of people living with HIV/AIDS in Eastern Europe, an estimated 860,000. There are increasing concerns about the spread of the pandemic in Asia as well, particularly China and India, the two other most populated regions in the world. Like Russia, they are considered part of the pandemic's next wave and despite having relatively low percentages of their population infected with HIV today the pandemic could expand significantly over the next decade if no changes are made. Researchers projected in the same May 2006 report mentioned above that by 2025, **31 million in India** and **18 million in China could die from AIDS** if infection rates don't drop. India already has the second highest number of people estimated to be living with HIV/AIDS in the world (5.1 million).

Also, approximately 11 of every 1,000 adults (ages 15 to 49) are HIV infected and **25 million children are projected to be orphans by 2010** because of AIDS.

AIDS/HIV Facts, Aids.com, *"Sharing Hope and Providing Knowledge"*

Sub-Saharan Africa

Sub-Saharan Africa has just over 10% of the world's population, but is home to more than 60% of all people living with HIV — **25.8 million.**

In 2005, an estimated 3.2 million people in the region became newly infected, while

2.4 million adults and children died of AIDS.

Asia

In 2005, some 8.3 million people were living with HIV in Asia, including 1.1 million people who became newly infected in the past year. **AIDS claimed some 520,000 lives in 2005.**

Eastern Europe and Central Asia

The number of people living with HIV in Eastern Europe and Central Asia reached an estimated 1.6 million in 2005.

Around **62,000 adults and children died of AIDS-related illnesses in 2005** and some 270,000 people were newly infected with HIV. Around 75% of the reported infections between 2000 and 2004 were in people younger than 30 years (in Western Europe, the corresponding figure was 33%).

Caribbean

The AIDS pandemic claimed an estimated 24,000 lives in the Caribbean **in 2005,** making it the leading cause of death among adults aged 15-44 years.

A total of 300,000 people are currently living with HIV in the region, including 30,000 people who became infected in 2005.

Latin America

The number of people living with HIV in Latin America has risen to an estimated 1.8 million.

In 2005, approximately 66,000 people died of AIDS, and 200,000 were newly infected. Among young people 15–24 years of age, an estimated 0.4% of women and 0.6% men were living with HIV in 2005.

Western and Central Europe

The number of people living with HIV in Western and Central Europe rose to more than 900,000 in **2005,** with approximately 23,000 people having acquired HIV in the past year.

Wide availability of antiretroviral therapy has helped keep **AIDS deaths** comparatively low, **at about 14,000 in 2005**.

Middle East and North Africa

The advance of AIDS in the Middle East and North Africa has continued with latest estimates showing that 67,000 people became infected with HIV in 2005.

Approximately 510,000 people are living with HIV in the region. **An estimated 58,000 adults and children died of AIDS-related illnesses in 2005.**

Oceania

An estimated 74,000 people in Oceania are living with HIV. Although **less than 4,000 people are believed to have died of AIDS in 2005**, about 8,200 are thought to have become newly infected with HIV.

Among young people 15–24 years of age, an estimated 1.2% of women and 0.4% of men were living with HIV in 2005.

Source: **UNAIDS** (United Nations). *UNAIDS/WHO estimates are based on all available data, including surveys of pregnant women, population-based surveys, and other surveillance information. UNAIDS views such information as complementary and useful in helping to estimate the number of people living with HIV in a country.*

(Please reference Exhibits on following pages for other basic local, national and international statistical information).

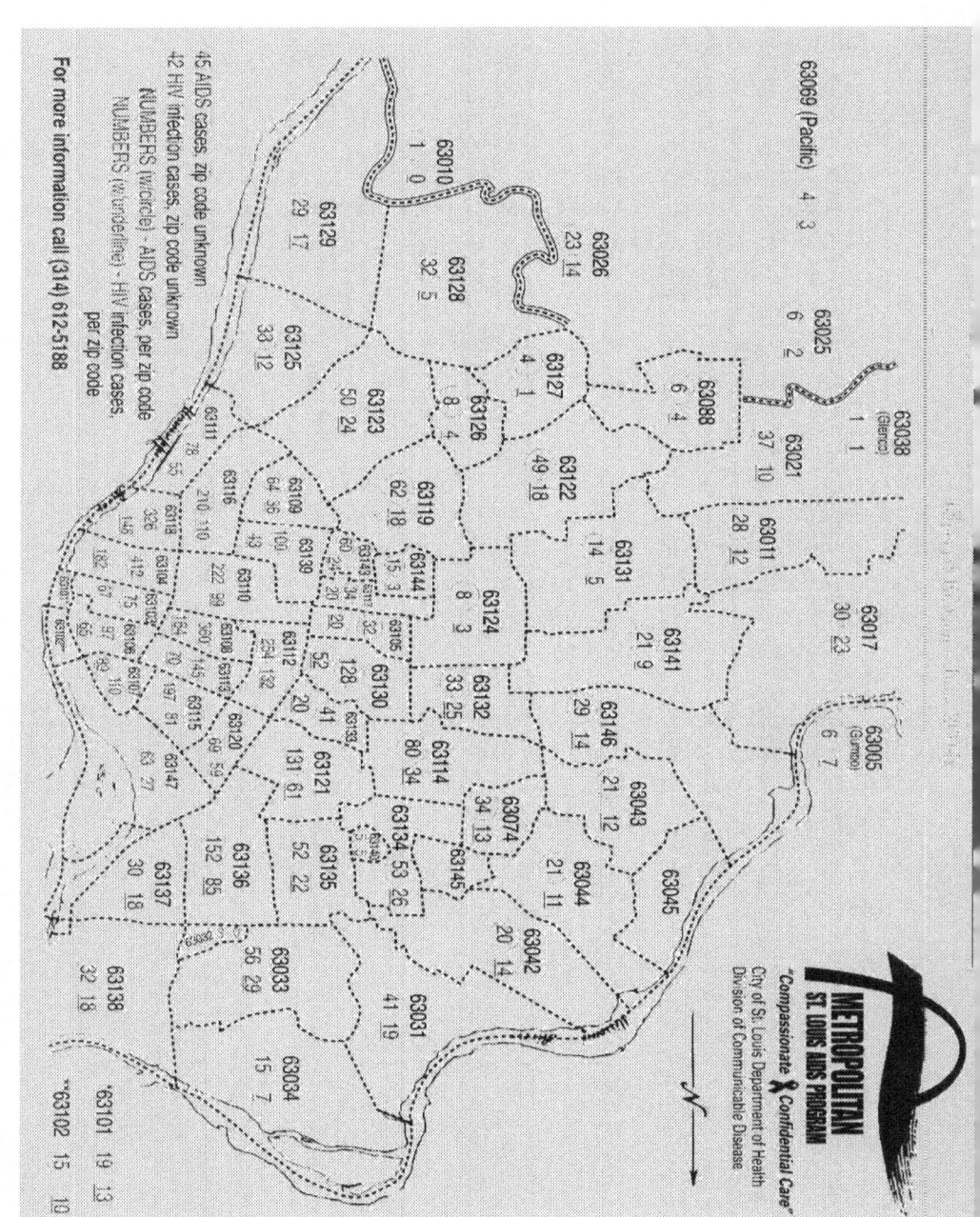

63069 (Pacific) 4 3

45 AIDS cases, zip code unknown
42 HIV infection cases, zip code unknown
NUMBERS (w/circle) - AIDS cases, per zip code
NUMBERS (w/underline) - HIV infection cases,
per zip code

For more information call (314) 612-5188

63010 1 0
63129 29 17
63128 32 5
63026 23 14
63025 6 2
63038 (Glencoe) 1 1
63125 38 12
63123 50 24
63126 8 4
63127 4 1
63088 6 4
63021 37 10
63122 49 18
63011 28 12
63017 30 23
63005 (Gumbo) 6 7

63111 78 55
63118 336
63116 210 110
63109 64 36
63119 62 18
63108 145
63104 412
63139 43 100
63110 222 99
63143 15 3
63144 26 20
63131 14 5
63141 21 9
63146 29 14
63043 21 12

63105 360
63115 70 46
63106 188 110
63112 254 132
63120 145
63147 63 77
63107 197 91
63133 69 50
63130 128
63124 8 3
63132 33 25
63114 80 34
63074 34 13
63044 21 11

63121 52 20
63134 53 26
63135 52 22
63145 21 11
63045

63137 30 18
63136 152 85
63042 20 14

63138 32 18
63033 56 29
63031 41 19

63034 15 7
63102 15 10
63101 19 13

METROPOLITAN
ST. LOUIS AIDS PROGRAM
"Compassionate & Confidential Care"
City of St. Louis Department of Health
Division of Communicable Disease

N →

- 24 -

The City of St. Louis Department of Health's HIV/AIDS Surveillance Unit reports that the Metropolitan St. Louis Statistics are:

- African American men represent 42% of the reported HIV cases among men

- African American men represent 39% of the reported AIDS cases among men

- African American men represent 67% of the total combined reported HIV/AIDS cases among men

- African American women represent 74% of the reported HIV cases among women

- African American women represent 68% of the reported AIDS cases among women

- African American women represent 80% of the total combined reported HIV/AIDS cases among women

- African American youth (13 – 25 years old) represent 74% of the reported HIV cases among youth

- African American youth represent 66% of the reported AIDS cases among youth

- African American youth represent 71% of the combined reported HIV/AIDS cases among youth

- African American persons over the age of 55 represent 55% of the reported HIV cases of persons over the age of 55

- African American persons over the age of 55 represent 41% of the reported AIDS cases of persons over the age of 55

- African American persons over the age of 55 represent 43% of reported cases of HIV/AIDS in persons over the age of 55

Area of residence	7/1995-6/1996	7/1996-6/1997	7/1997-6/1998	7/1998-6/1999	7/1999-6/2000	7/2000-6/2001	7/2001-6/2002	7/2002-6/2003	7/2003-6/2004	7/2004-6/2005
Alabama	625	497	581	438	446	421	373	482	458	503
Alaska	37	41	37	24	12	39	18	33	27	55
Arizona	634	508	504	670	610	464	493	632	656	625
Arkansas	246	223	208	172	178	175	237	170	223	152
California	10,020	7,762	6,001	5,327	4,397	4,371	3,985	4,917	5,137	4,419
Colorado	586	419	292	321	283	298	286	372	300	387
Connecticut	1,468	1,153	863	589	619	492	635	574	815	682
Delaware	303	249	157	167	189	231	240	211	162	127
District of Columbia	1,033	1,139	882	898	904	886	684	1,106	820	1,104
Florida	7,263	6,292	5,024	5,170	4,522	4,705	4,560	4,655	5,395	5,661
Georgia	2,323	1,954	1,274	1,494	1,215	1,282	1,704	1,355	1,967	1,860
Hawaii	191	137	120	122	118	63	140	121	93	151
Idaho	39	43	38	27	25	19	18	29	21	20
Illinois	2,084	1,898	1,696	1,225	1,950	1,187	1,560	2,166	1,521	1,829
Indiana	601	520	458	326	348	332	462	466	441	423
Iowa	116	98	67	75	61	85	86	81	69	68
Kansas	218	155	126	129	142	91	90	76	133	117
Kentucky	296	374	295	288	230	279	269	233	241	280
Louisiana	1,294	1,169	1,005	846	668	743	864	1,050	1,182	868
Maine	68	52	40	39	62	39	45	44	31	57
Maryland	2,171	2,056	1,551	1,552	1,330	1,559	1,978	1,606	1,541	1,577
Massachusetts	1,206	1,018	696	1,160	1,367	763	691	752	657	701
Michigan	988	886	761	681	571	742	634	740	672	655
Minnesota	318	241	173	200	189	173	141	164	193	249
Mississippi	390	416	337	405	383	438	345	449	522	482
Missouri	785	647	503	439	444	410	324	430	384	424
Montana	29	39	32	18	18	14	9	15	6	7
Nebraska	94	96	71	69	59	83	64	69	49	66
Nevada	412	407	417	240	273	221	257	302	279	337
New Hampshire	95	67	50	45	35	27	43	35	46	36
New Jersey	3,828	3,596	2,375	1,945	1,740	1,762	1,557	1,500	1,444	1,637
New Mexico	102	205	198	111	119	102	129	86	148	151
New York	12,787	11,901	10,830	7,298	6,631	5,140	7,567	6,590	7,102	7,842
North Carolina	825	838	773	751	688	692	939	1,229	784	1,335
North Dakota	10	9	11	5	5	3	3	3	15	9
Ohio	1,042	899	754	565	579	488	673	724	633	751
Oklahoma	258	264	269	162	213	283	242	190	188	277
Oregon	451	329	208	182	205	205	282	256	262	288
Pennsylvania	2,150	1,996	1,762	1,661	1,519	1,546	1,998	1,673	1,704	1,584
Puerto Rico	1,987	2,075	1,909	1,390	950	1,346	1,230	1,155	652	1,242
Rhode Island	171	181	125	110	88	97	107	104	114	130
South Carolina	896	755	726	918	747	680	753	797	744	77
South Dakota	16	10	16	17	8	23	8	14	14	16
Tennessee	850	755	649	725	599	698	688	820	781	822
Texas	4,158	4,533	4,217	3,494	2,397	2,587	2,767	2,861	3,909	3,091
Utah	187	147	136	146	131	140	94	86	73	81
Vermont	36	30	18	15	26	28	21	10	23	8
Virgin Islands	31	49	59	33	41	16	63	36	23	24
Virginia	1,419	1,179	924	825	855	917	884	808	731	774
Washington	730	704	493	357	423	480	476	435	518	461
West Virginia	135	102	116	58	61	71	90	78	73	99
Wisconsin	317	243	214	176	160	194	219	183	163	173
Wyoming	13	18	5	7	16	5	8	11	9	14

Centers for Disease Control and Prevention, 1600 Clifton Rd. Atlanta, GA 30333, U.S.A.
Tel. (404) 639-3311 / Public Inquiries (404) 639-3534 / (800) 311-3435

Estimated Number of Adults and Children Newly Infected with HIV During 2004

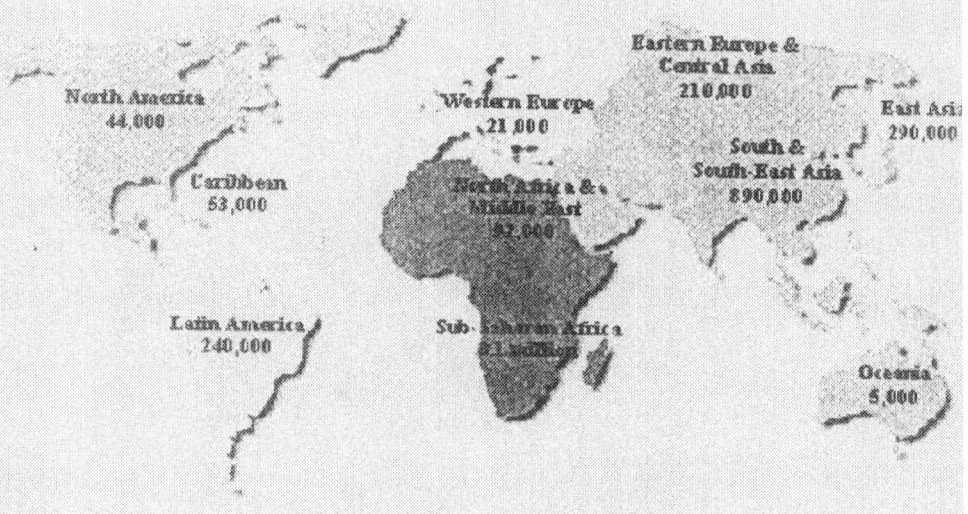

North America
44,000

Western Europe
21,000

Eastern Europe &
Central Asia
210,000

East Asia
290,000

Caribbein
53,000

North Africa & &
Middle East
92,000

South &
South-East Asia
890,000

Latin America
240,000

Sub-Saharan Africa
3.1 million

Oceania
5,000

Total: 4.9 million
Source: UNAIDS

Information Source: AIDS.com: HIV/AIDS Facts

Adults and Children Estimated to be Living
with HIV as of 2004

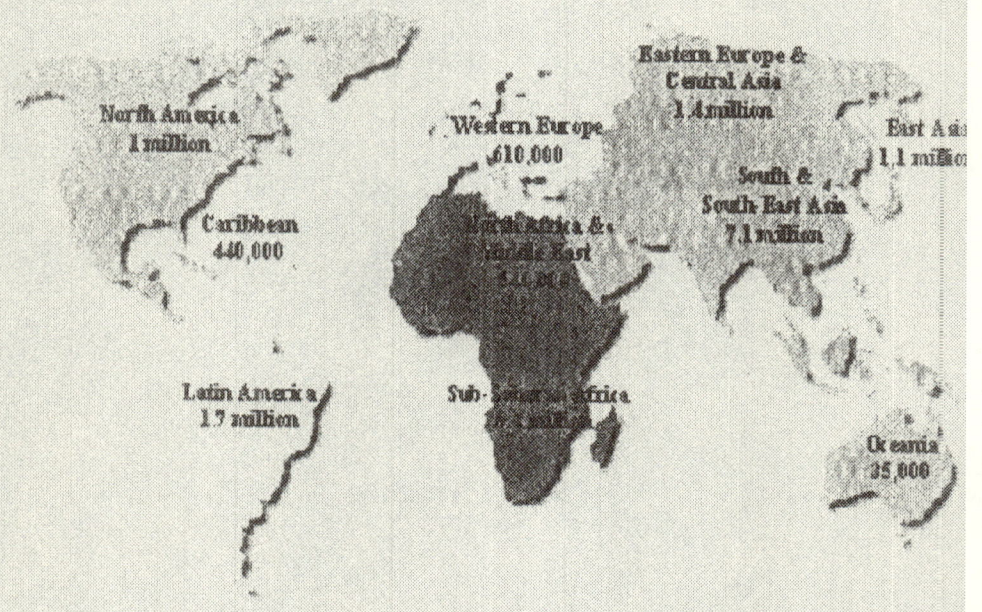

Total 39.4 million
Source: UNAIDS

Information Source: AIDS.com: HIV/AIDS Facts

Estimated Adult and Child Deaths from AIDS During 2004

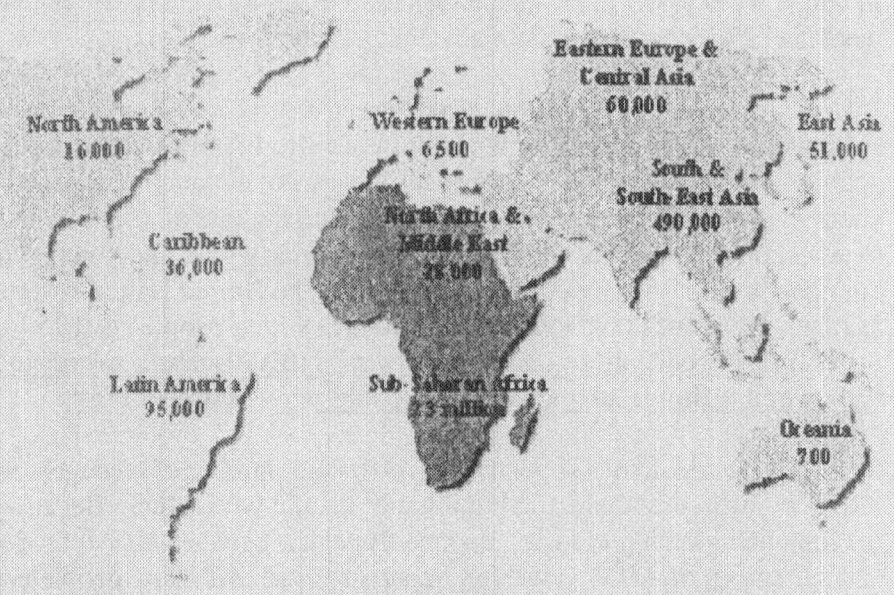

North America
16,000

Caribbean
36,000

Latin America
95,000

Western Europe
6,500

North Africa &
Middle East
28,000

Sub-Saharan Africa
2.3 million

Eastern Europe &
Central Asia
60,000

South &
South East Asia
490,000

East Asia
51,000

Oceania
700

Total: 3.1 million
Source: UNAIDS

United States Statistics

- At least 40,000 new HIV infections per year
- 1 million United States residents currently living with HIV, 25% are unaware of their infection
- Over 16,000 AIDS related deaths in 2004

Information Source: AIDS.com: HIV/AIDS Facts

Impact of HIV/AIDS on Youth Population

The potential impact of HIV among teenagers is great. Some teens feel safe and invulnerable because they may not have seen anyone their age or otherwise with AIDS. Many teens experiment with drugs, alcohol and sex, which puts them at a much greater risk. Taking risks is a common way in which teens assert their independence. They may use sexual behavior to meet needs for friendship, intimacy and peer approval.

A disease which was once considered a surefire, automatic death sentence is now seldom thought about in the area of curtailing sexual activity amongst our youth. As a result, many are not at all concerned about the consequences of HIV and AIDS, and the rate of youth infection is skyrocketing. Teens and young adults, particularly girls and young women, continue to be at the center of the epidemic. The United Nations estimates as many as half of all new infections occur in young people aged 15 to 24. Sadly, **indifference and unconcern towards this disease is occurring at a time when intimate sexual behavior could prove fatal**.

Current statistics show a relatively small number of teenagers with AIDS, compared with the total number of people with AIDS. Because of the long incubation period (as much as 10 years) between HIV infection and symptoms of AIDS, however, experts believe that many people now in their twenties with AIDS (almost 20 percent of all AIDS cases) became infected when they were teenagers. Thus, current AIDS statistics do not give an accurate picture of HIV infection among teenagers, which may prove devastating.

Youth today live in an extremely sexually charged culture. They see it everywhere they turn and it launches a violent attack on impressionable young minds. When I talk with teens about HIV/AIDS, I attempt to drive home the point that if they become sexually active in this current disease-saturated society, they are playing Russian Roulette with their lives. It amounts to taking a loaded gun, placing it to their temple and pulling the trigger – you may get the bullet and then you may not – but why take such a dangerous chance?

As we have seen, HIV/AIDS does not discriminate. It is devastating to people of all ages, genders, races, religions and nationalities regardless if you are gay, straight, a drug user or not. It can reach you in the most innocent of ways and *that's* what makes the disease so very dangerous. You cannot look at a person and tell whether they have AIDS or not. The gaunt, ashen, sickly look of yesteryear's AIDS is no more. AIDS looks like *you* – and it looks like *me*. AIDS is now *beautiful*. It is buff, muscular and attractive. The methods by which to get AIDS have been made glamorous. But after 25 years in this modern age of medicine and technology, there is *still* no cure. This disease *can be prevented,* however, through (1) self-control, (2) abandoning risky behaviors, (3) education and (4) awareness.

In the past, medical science has provided relief for man's promiscuous indiscretions, thereby alleviating some of the physical consequences. As a result, man has heedlessly, callously thrown caution to the four winds and indulged his every lustful passion. And though while new drug therapies make living with HIV more of a reality than ever before, millions continue to die, either because they cannot afford these life-extending drugs, they are in denial and refuse to begin treatment, or because they've developed a new form of AIDS that is non-responsive to existing drug therapies.

Nearly all of the currently approved medicines fall into one of three classes. When a patient's HIV develops resistance to any one drug, it typically has a head start on resisting other drugs from that class, too. Drug resistance normally brews slowly in an individual's body, as the internal tug of war between virus and medicines goes on over years. But it's also possible to become infected with a smarter HIV right from the start, from someone who had already exhausted some medicine's potential (Steven J. Fallon, Ph.D., *"It's the Best Time to Get HIV, and the Worst,"* May/June 2005).

The burden of side effects and complex dosing schedules, all while under the shock of one's new HIV status, is often overwhelming. Many patients miss doses of their medicines, triggering more dangerous strains of HIV to grow in their bodies (Steven J. Fallon, Ph.D., *"It's the Best Time to Get HIV, and the Worst,"* May/June 2005).

The sad reality is that this disease has been so glamorized by the media and new drugs have made it appear that people living with HIV live relatively normal lives that **many others will die because they don't**

believe AIDS is still a deadly disease. Even in America, many die every day from heart attacks, strokes, kidney failure, certain cancers and other ailments – *caused by* **but not attributed to HIV/AIDS-related infection**. More and more we hear about young people in their teens, 20s, 30s, etc., dying from ailments that were previously only found in much older people.

Recent breakthroughs in drug treatment, however, means the overwhelming fear of the late 1980s has vanished – and with it, life-saving, precautionary measures. Today, people in many countries, including the United States, have seen people live symptom-free for years with an HIV-positive diagnosis (TIME Magazine, *AIDS from the Front*, July 2002). The general but unfortunate mind-set of many young people is that "I'm going to die from something anyway. I may as well *ENJOY!*" In 2005 HIV/AIDS testing was performed in one popular St. Louis county school. **A mind-numbing over 80% of the students tested, were positive**...

Another sad reality is the politics involved in getting medicines to the people who desperately need them but cannot afford the treatment therapies. The big problem is money for research and prevention programs, and who should provide the funding. Many activists have argued that the richest nations, including the United States, have shown a lack of commitment to fighting the spread of HIV and AIDS, in not providing a means of affordable treatment.

In his State of the Union address (February 1, 2006), President Bush said, "More than a million Americans live with HIV, and half of all AIDS cases occur among Blacks" (*United Press International*, 2/1). Bush said he would lead a nationwide effort, in which he would work to "deliver rapid HIV tests to millions, end the stigma of AIDS and come closer to the day when there are no new [HIV cases] in America." Globally, Bush said the United States must "take the offensive by encouraging economic progress and fighting disease," including HIV/AIDS (*United Press International*, 2/1).

President Bush called on Congress to reauthorize the Ryan White CARE Act and increase funding for states to eliminate waiting lists for HIV/AIDS-related medications in the U.S. *United Press International*, February 1, 2006. The CARE Act, which expired Sept. 30, 2005, provides funding for care and services to HIV-positive people in the U.S. Twenty-one state **AIDS Drug Assistance Programs** (ADAP) either have implemented waiting lists or other cost-containment measures or are considering such measures. ADAPs are federal- and state-funded programs that provide HIV/AIDS-related medications to low-income, uninsured and underinsured HIV-positive individuals (*Kaiser Daily HIV/AIDS Report*, 12/8/05).

AIDS Project Los Angeles "welcomed" Bush's push for the reauthorization of the CARE Act. However, Executive Director Craig Thompson said, "Bush has had six years to appropriate funding to end waiting lists for life-saving HIV/AIDS medications in this country. It is hard not to be skeptical when there is no will behind the words." Thompson also said that Bush's proposal to make rapid HIV tests more widely available and end the stigma surrounding HIV/AIDS will "cost billions," adding, "We will never 'prevent, treat and defeat' domestic AIDS at the rate we're going" (APLA release, 1/31).

~~~~~~~~~~~~~~~~~~~~

If you have been paying the least bit of attention to the statistics and dates, you have noticed that some of the estimates are from 2003 and 2004. *These estimates are the most current available from all major surveillance sources.* **The Center for Disease Control (CDC) in Atlanta is the nation's ultimate resource and *the* last word for statistical information on every disease from AIDS to TB** to the bird flu. **Yet, on the 2004-2005 "AIDS Cases by State" exhibit in this book, the CDC shows that the total number of AIDS cases in the entire state of Missouri is 424.** *However,* **for the St. Louis metropolitan area *alone* and during the same 2004-2005 period the "HIV/AIDS Surveillance Newsletter" shows 412 AIDS infections *in only one zip code*: 63104**! It is logical to assume that if such statistical disparities exist between the CDC and *this* state, **there are gross disparities in statistical AIDS data all *across the nation*!**

The truth of the matter is that it is virtually *impossible* to know the more precise numbers due to the fact a great many of the **safety nets previously utilized are no longer in place**. For instance, mandatory blood testing prior to marriage in Missouri is no longer a requirement (this was discovered when my daughter was about to wed). Mandatory blood testing was a very effective means of tracking disease, which would set off a chain-reaction of information being passed to the appropriate local and national health agencies. Local agencies do not list statistical data on their websites, or through any other means. Some of these agencies don't even *have* a website.

The part that scares me is that only *once a year* is vital statistical information distributed to the general public, usually during the "Week of Prayer for the Healing of AIDS" in black churches. After that week, no mention is ever made again of HIV/AIDS publicly. In St. Louis (2006), the "*Week* of Prayer" was cut to only *four days* of prayer – with each year receiving less and less participation, as if a cure for AIDS has been found. **If in 2004, 1 in 10 Americans** (not *black* Americans, not *white* Americans – but *Americans*) *50 and above (!!!)* **were HIV/AIDS positive, what are the stats in 2006?** If **1 in 50** black men were HIV/AIDS positive in 2004, what are the stats in 2006 – 1 in 35, 1 in 30? One thing is certain: stats are not improving but *worsening*. Across the board, figures are *accelerating*, not decreasing, while there is much less concern now than ever...

It is apparent that **there is a serious breakdown in the number of reporting sites that could provide closer-to-actual statistics**. However, one frightening detail stands out: **whatever statistical information these reporting sites are prepared with are only of the number of *known* cases that have been *reported*.** There are *many* people, however, who are infected and are *aware* of their HIV-positive but have not reported their status to an agency and continue to be sexually active. There are also those that are infected but *unaware* of their status, simply because they have failed to be tested. They, too, are sexually active. In any event, it may very well be that the numbers we *don't know* by far exceed the numbers that have been reported. The fact is -- whether their status is known or unknown -- **there are those who are committing *suicide, homicide and genocide*** simply by being sexually active in this diseased-saturated society.

An individual's right to privacy has become the larger issue in many states. In most states, **if two people are married and one of them becomes infected after marriage, the doctor is prohibited by law from telling the spouse of the infected partner!** In New York City, the Health Commissioner recently called for changing state regulations on HIV/AIDS testing services to allow health officials to "more aggressively test people for HIV/AIDS," as well as to allow officials to use information they already collect on HIV-positive people. It was proposed in order to meet the city mayor's goal of reducing AIDS-related deaths by more than 40%.

New York City and the state collect data about HIV-positive people, but as in many other states, *current laws* prevent health officials from contacting patients or their physicians about treatment. "We know people are dying and we are prohibited by law from lifting a finger to try and help," the Health Commissioner stated.

Perhaps even more importantly, the Health Commissioner also called for "making testing for the virus a routine part of medical care" and suggested requiring only verbal consent for HIV/AIDS testing services, rather than both written and verbal, and is in no way proposing mandatory testing or treatment." Other city officials are worried this may cause a violation of privacy issues.

Granted, **very few who live moral lives get AIDS**. However, one of the principal concerns regarding AIDS, and a major reason for writing this book is although abstinence is the *only sure way* of not contracting AIDS or any other STD, there are many, *many* cases where complete innocents are involved. For example, in *marriage* in which abstinence is not a practical solution, one marriage mate may be moral but the other mate may be immoral and infected with AIDS and thus pass on the disease to the innocent mate. In this present society, it happens far more often than we are prepared to admit. Of course, an innocent mate who suspects the other of immorality or drug abuse has the right to take protective steps. The innocent victim is _not_ required to commit suicide!

Shoko Nagaya of the health ministry in Toyko advised: "Know your partner." But in the current sexual climate in which we live, is it even *possible* to 'know your partner'? The Tokyo newspaper Asahi Shimbun quotes health officials as saying: "If you are leading an ordinary life, you will not contract the disease. So there is no reason to be inordinately worried about the disease. But if you want to 'fool around,' do so at your own risk, the risk of committing suicide."

Today, women represent 48% of all adults living with HIV/AIDS, and the number of women living with the disease has increased globally. Gender inequalities in social and economic status and in access to prevention and care services increase women's vulnerability to HIV infection. Sexual abuse and violence may also increase women's risk and women, especially young women, are biologically more susceptible to HIV infection than men (UNAIDS, *2006 AIDS Epidemic Update, December 2006*).

One young lady, Joyce Russ*, could have done little to protect herself against infection. Her abusive husband was infected before their marriage, and they were married at a time when the pandemic and HIV testing were in their early stages. However, now HIV testing has become a routine procedure. Even though mandatory blood testing is no longer required for marriage, it is wise to test *even before* engagement.

Testing may help to protect an innocent mate in cases of infidelity and adultery. Since HIV might not show up on a test until up to six months after infection, *several* tests might be necessary. Joyce's advice: "Know your marriage partner *before* you marry them. A wrong choice can cost you dearly, even life itself."

*Name changed to protect privacy

~~~~~~~~~~~~~~~~~~

What many people don't know, or fail to comprehend – and not just *teenagers* – is the complete probability of STD infection by 'degrees of association'. **The basic truth is that when you have sex with someone, you are also having sex with everyone else your partner has been with.** (*English,* please?) What this means is: if you are having sex with someone, and *that* person has had sex with say five or six other people, *you* are essentially having sex with *all* of them! Not only that, you are also having sex *with every partner* the five or six others had sex with! When you think about it, the numbers are staggering. Just *one act* of sexual intercourse or oral sex could expose you to countless other people and *their* sexually transmitted diseases and infections. If you are sexually active today ask yourself: What are my odds of contracting some type of STD? Answer: nearly 100%... **Having sex in this present culture with anyone other than a *faithful* marriage mate is like playing Russian Roulette: *eventually* you're going to catch that bullet...**

Whenever a new disease comes along, there is always speculation about where it came from and how it got started. The truth is that HIV appears to have spread to humans from monkeys. The same virus in monkeys is called SIV, for *Simian Immunodeficiency Virus*. HIV-1 – the strain most common in Central and Southern Africa, the United States and the rest of the world – seems to have come from chimpanzees.

HIV-2 – the strain found in West Africa – seems to have come from the sooty mangabey monkey. HIV is not the only virus that has spread to humans from animals – researchers suspect that SARS may have spread to humans from the civet cat. And many types of flu are thought to have originated in chickens.

In the United States, doctors in Los Angeles and New York reported unusual cases of Pneumocystis carinii pneumonia and Kaposi's sarcoma in 1981. The Centers for Disease Control and Prevention (CDC) then began tracking a growing number of young men, women and babies who suffered from these illnesses and whose immune systems were nearly destroyed. Their condition was not referred to as "AIDS," however, until late 1982. Scientists have found evidence that the disease existed in the world for some years before it was recognized in 1981.

A disease is considered *epidemic* when it is contained on a local level. However, when the disease spreads nationally and internationally, it is categorized as *pandemic*.

AIDS is caused by **HIV,** or **H**uman **I**mmunodeficiency **V**irus. By killing or damaging cells of the body's immune system, HIV progressively destroys the body's ability to fight infections and certain forms of cancer. People diagnosed with AIDS may get life-threatening diseases called 'opportunistic infections,' which are caused by microbes, such as, viruses or bacteria that usually do not make healthy people sick.

I have been told by health professionals that the disease is not what kills – the damage that is done by the disease within a person's body is what actually kills. In other words, you may hear of a 20-year old dying from a massive heart attack, or stroke, or kidney failure, or certain kinds of cancer due to the disease's presence in the body. The cause of death is not ruled to be 'death by HIV/AIDS' but rather to the failure of whatever vital organ the disease has attacked. This is much less stigmatic than attributing the cause of death to HIV/AIDS. As I previously stated, *privacy – **not** the disease – is the larger issue in America*…

Transmission

HIV is spread most commonly by having unprotected sex with an infected partner. The virus can enter the body through the lining of the vagina, vulva, penis, anus, rectum, or mouth during sex. HIV can infect anyone who practices risky behaviors, such as:

- Having sexual contact, including oral, with an infected person
- Having sexual contact with someone whose HIV status is unknown
- Sharing drug needles or syringes

HIV is also spread through contact with infected blood. Before donated blood was screened for evidence of infection and before heat-treating techniques were developed to destroy HIV in blood products, HIV was transmitted through transfusions of contaminated blood or blood components. Today, however, **the risk of getting HIV from transfusions is small due to current blood-screening** and heat treatment practices.

Scientists have found no evidence that HIV is spread through sweat, tears, urine, or feces. Also, researchers have found no evidence that the virus is spread by contact with saliva. However, the lining of the mouth *can* be infected by HIV and instances of HIV transmission through oral intercourse have been reported.

Studies have clearly shown that HIV is *not* spread through casual contact such as the sharing of eating utensils, food, towels and bedding, swimming pools, telephones or toilet seats. HIV is also *not* spread by mosquitoes, bedbugs or other blood-sucking, biting insects.

If you have a sexually transmitted infection (STI), such as, syphilis, genital herpes, chlamydial infection, gonorrhea, or bacterial vaginosis, you may be more susceptible to getting HIV infection during sex with an infected partner.

Early Symptoms of HIV Infection

Symptoms are not immediately noticed when a person first becomes infected with HIV. There may be an occasional **flu-like illness** within a month or two after exposure to the virus. This illness **may include fever, a constant headache, unusual tiredness, and enlarged lymph nodes, which can be easily felt in the neck and groin areas**.

These symptoms usually disappear within a week to a month and are often mistaken for other, less serious viral infections. During this period, people are very infectious and HIV is present in large quantities in genital fluids. More persistent or severe symptoms may not appear for 10 years or more after HIV first enters the body in adults, or within 2 years in children born with HIV infection. This period of "asymptomatic" infection varies in each individual. Some people may begin to have symptoms within just a few months, while others may be completely symptom-free for many years.

Even during the symptom-free period, the disease is actively at work – multiplying, infecting, and killing cells of the immune system. The virus can also hide within infected cells and lay dormant.

As the immune system weakens, a variety of complications start to take over. For many people, the first signs of infection are enlarged lymph nodes or swollen glands that may be enlarged for more than three months. Other symptoms that are often experienced months to years before the onset of AIDS include:

- Lack of energy
- Weight loss
- Frequent fevers and sweats
- Persistent or frequent yeast infections (oral or vaginal)
- Persistent skin rashes or flaky skin
- Pelvic inflammatory disease in women that does not respond to treatment
- Short-term memory loss
- Diarrhea that lasts for more than a week

- Pelvic inflammatory disease in women that does not respond to treatment
- Dry cough
- Pneumonia
- White spots or unusual blemishes on the tongue, in the mouth, or in the throat

Some people develop frequent and severe herpes infections that cause mouth, genital, or anal sores, or a painful nerve disease called shingles. Children may grow more slowly than others, or be sick a great deal.

Symptoms of AIDS (Acquired Immunodeficiency Syndrome) Infections

The Center for Disease Control (CDC) developed official criteria for the definition of AIDS and is responsible for tracking the spread of AIDS in the United States. **The CDC's definition of AIDS includes all HIV-infected people who have fewer than 200 CD4+ T cells per cubic millimeter of blood.** (Healthy adults usually have CD4+ T-cell counts of 1,000 or more). In addition, the definition, the definition includes 26 clinical conditions that affect people with advanced HIV disease.

Most of these conditions are "opportunistic infections" that generally do not affect normal, healthy people. In people with AIDS, however, these infections are often severe and sometimes fatal because the immune system is so ravaged by HIV that the body cannot fight off certain viruses, bacteria and other microbes. Also, it must be noted that **the disease has the potential to attack *other* major organs** of a person's body, **such as, the heart, brain, kidneys, lungs**, etc., establishing infections in those in advanced stages of the disease.

Symptoms of opportunistic infections common in people with AIDS include coughing, shortness of breath, lack of coordination, fever, severe and persistent diarrhea, vomiting, severe headaches, nausea, abdominal cramps, extreme fatigue, weight loss, vision loss, confusion, forgetfulness, seizures and coma.

People with AIDS are also prone to developing various cancers, such as, Kaposi's sarcoma and cervical cancer, or cancers of the immune and lymph systems, known as lymphomas. **It is entirely possible for the disease to create cancer in any portion of your body containing lymph nodes:** neck, stomach, groin and underarms.

Many people are so debilitated by the symptoms of AIDS that they cannot hold a steady job nor do common household chores. Other people with AIDS may experience phases of intense life-threatening illness, followed by phases in which they function normally.

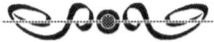

The Crisis

<u>Source References</u>

- *"Working Towards Independence,"* [Encourage Abstinence and Prevent Teen Pregnancy], United States Government, February 2002
- *"The Truth about STDs"*, Sexuality Information and Education Council of the United States, March 2003
- Stanley Falkow, *"Who Speaks for the Microbes?,"* Stanford University School of Medicine, Stanford, California, USA
- David H. Martin, *"Medical Clinics of North America"*, W.B. Saunders Company; Harcourt Brace Jovanovich, Inc., Nov. 1990
- Dr. Stuart Levy, *"The Antibiotic Paradox: How the Miracle Drugs Are Destroying the Miracle"*
- Time Magazine, *AIDS: Report from the Front*
- Glynn M., Rhodes P. Estimated HIV prevalence in the United States at the end of 2003. *National HIV Prevention Conference; June 2005; Atlanta. Abstract 595*
- CDC HIV/AIDS Surveillance Report: *HIV Infection and AIDS in the United States*, 2003
- U.S. Dept. of Health and Human Services, *National Institute of Allergy and Infectious Diseases,* March 2005
- American International AIDS Foundation, 2006
- Source: *UNAIDS* (United Nations)
- Santora, *New York Times*, February 2, 2006
- HIV *Positive!*, "HIV 101," February/March 2004
- *Nature*, 1998; vol. 391, no. 5. *"An African HIV 1 Sequence from 1959 and the Implications for the Origin of the Pandemic."* Letters to Nature. Zhu, 7:, et al.
- DeVita, V., Jr., et al., eds. *AIDS: Etiology, Diagnosis, Treatment and Prevention*, 4th ed. 1997.
- Centers for Disease Control and Prevention. *MMWR*, 1981; vol. 30, no. 21. *"Pneumocystis* Pneumonia -- Los Angeles."
- KnowHIV/AIDS: *"Get The Facts Statistics"*
- American Red Cross, "Health & Safety Services – *HIV/AIDS Facts*", November 2001.

RISK FACTORS AMONG BLACKS

Even though *all* minority populations are disproportionately affected by the HIV/AIDS pandemic, it is a *severe* health crisis for Blacks. Please pay close attention to the statistical data. The disease is growing at an astonishing rate among minority populations and is a **leading killer of Blacks ages 25 to 44.** According to the Centers for Disease Control and Prevention (CDC), AIDS affects nearly *seven times* more Blacks and *three times* more Hispanics than whites. In recent years, an increasing number of Black women and children are being affected by HIV/AIDS. In 2003, two-thirds of United States AIDS cases in both women and children were among Blacks.

HIV/AIDS and Blacks

In 2001, HIV/AIDS was among the top three (3) causes of death for Black men aged 25–54 years and among the top four (4) causes of death for Black women aged 20–54 years. It was the number 1 cause of death for Black women aged 25–34 years.

HIV/AIDS Statistics

Cumulative Effects of HIV/AIDS (through 2003)

According to the 2000 census, Blacks make up 12.3% of the United States population. However, they have accounted for 368,169 (40%) of the 929,985 estimated AIDS cases diagnosed since the pandemic began.

- By the end of December 2003, an estimated 195,891 Blacks with AIDS had died.
- Of persons given a diagnosis of AIDS since 1995, a smaller proportion of Blacks (60%) were alive after 9 years compared with American Indians and Alaska Natives (64%), Hispanics (68%), whites (70%), and Asians and Pacific Islanders (77%).
- During 2000–2005, HIV rates for Black females were 23 times the rates for white females and 5 times the rates for Hispanic females; they also exceeded the rates for males of all races/ethnicities other than Blacks. Rates for Black males were 7 times those for white males and 3 times those for Hispanic males.

AIDS in 2003

- The rate of AIDS diagnoses for Blacks was almost 10 times the rate for whites and almost 3 times the rate for Hispanics. The rate of AIDS diagnoses for Black women was 25 times the rate for white women. The rate of AIDS diagnoses for Black men was 8 times the rate for white men.
- In the United States, 172,278 Blacks were living with AIDS. They accounted for 42% of all people in the United States living with AIDS.
- Of the 59 US children younger than 13 years of age who had a new AIDS diagnosis, 40 were Black.

HIV/AIDS in 2003

- Blacks accounted for 16,165 (50%) of the 32,048 estimated new HIV/AIDS diagnoses in the United States in the 32 states with confidential name-based HIV reporting.
- A study of people with a diagnosis of HIV infection found that 56% of late testers (that is, those who received an AIDS diagnosis within 1 year after their HIV diagnosis) were Black. Late testing represents missed opportunities for preventing and treating HIV infection.
- The leading cause of HIV infection among Black men was sexual contact with other men; the next leading causes were heterosexual contact and injection drug use.
- The leading cause of HIV infection among Black women was heterosexual contact; the next leading cause was injection drug use.
- Of the 90 infants reported as having HIV/ AIDS, 62 were Black.

~~~~~~~~~~~~~~~~~~~~

BARRIERS TO PREVENTION AMONG BLACKS

Race and ethnicity are not, by themselves, risk factors for HIV infection. However, Blacks are more likely to face challenges associated with risk for HIV infection, such as:

Partners at Risk

Black women are most likely to be infected with HIV as a result of sex with men. They may not be aware of their male partners' possible risks for HIV infection such as unprotected sex with multiple partners, bisexuality, or injection drug use. According to a recent study of HIV infected and non-infected Black men who have sex with men (MSM), approximately 20% of the study participants reported having had a female sex partner during the preceding 12 months. In another study of HIV-infected persons, 34% of Black MSM reported having had sex with women, even though only 6% of Black women reported having had sex with a bisexual man.

Substance Abuse

Injection drug use is the second leading cause of HIV infection for Black women and the third leading cause of HIV infection for Black men. In addition to being at risk from sharing needles, casual and chronic drug users are more likely to engage in high-risk behaviors, such as unprotected sex, when they are under the influence of drugs or alcohol. Drug use can also affect treatment success. A recent study of HIV-infected women found that drug users were less likely than nonusers to take their antiretroviral medicines exactly as prescribed.

Sexually Transmitted Diseases

The highest rates of sexually transmitted diseases (STDs) are those for Blacks. In 2003, Blacks were 20 times as likely as whites to have gonorrhea and 5.2 times as likely to have syphilis. Partly because of physical changes caused by STDs, including genital lesions that can serve as an entry point for HIV, the presence of certain STDs can increase one's chances of contracting HIV by 3- to 5-fold. Similarly, a person who is co-infected has a greater chance of spreading HIV to others.

Denial

Studies show that a significant number of Black MSM (men who have sex with men) identify themselves as heterosexual. As a result, they may not relate to prevention messages crafted for men who identify themselves as strictly homosexual. Also classified in this category are homo-thugs (younger set of bisexual males) and men on the DL (down-low), who more than likely have a female partner and children.

Socioeconomic Issues

Nearly 1 in 4 Blacks lives in poverty. Studies have found an association between higher AIDS incidence and lower income. The socioeconomic problems associated with poverty, including limited access to high-quality health care and HIV prevention education, directly or indirectly increase HIV risk. A recent study of HIV transmission among Black women in North Carolina found that women with HIV infection were more likely than non-infected women to be unemployed, receive public assistance have had 20 or more lifetime sexual partners, have a lifetime history of genital herpes infection, have used crack or cocaine, or have traded sex for drugs, money, or shelter.

~~~~~~~~~~~~~~~~~~~~

Perhaps the most frightening comment made in 2004 was made by the St. Louis City Health Commissioner during the "Week of Prayer for the Healing of AIDS", who stated that at the current rate of growth of HIV/AIDS infections within the African-American community, by mid-century there may be a model of a black male and female in the Smithsonian Institute – beside the dinosaur...

The reality of the plight of the black minority in America as it relates to HIV/AIDS infections and other health issues, places them in a far more precarious position than any other racial group – of even blacks in Africa. However, to this point, blacks in America have been unconvinced of the gravity of the out-of-control rate of HIV/AIDS' growth within their ethnic group, much less over the disease's ability to completely eradicate the race. The unfortunate truth about this way of thinking, however, is that it *does not* change the reality of the crisis: **HIV's overwhelming concentration** within the African-American community has the potential to carry an entire race of people the way of the dinosaur**. Let us take a look at how this is possible:

First of all, let us establish once and for all that Africa is a CONTINENT – America is only a COUNTRY. Africa is comprised of many, *many* countries, some of which are larger than America. **African-Americans' presence in the country comes to roughly 12.5 percent** of the population. Currently, **blacks make up 50%* of all people with HIV/AIDS in America** and **55%* of total** *new* **HIV/AIDS cases**. Considering the fact that the **African-American population is relatively small and the infection rate of HIV/AIDS is so high**, the sum total of the figures equal *disaster…*

*(Information with an asterisk (*) is based on known and reported HIV/AIDS cases in America, per the Center for Disease Control (CDC). **As a rule of thumb, there are more cases unknown and unreported than are***).

It must also be noted that aside from HIV's high infection rate within the black community, **the race has an array of *other* killer health issues**: diabetes, hypertension, heart disease, etc. This fact, **combined with unhealthy practices, addictions, risky behaviors and other STDs (some of which have the ability to cause sterilization in men), puts the perpetuation of the race in question past 50 more years.**

An October 2000 issue of the *Discover* magazine reported that **99% of all life** (human, animal, plant and sea life) **that ever existed on Earth is now extinct**. During the latter portion of 2006, a *60 Minutes* episode noted the polar bear is now endangered due to global warming – and projected the species would become extinct by the end of the century. However, if African-Americans do not *immediately* move towards improving overall health -- which includes eliminating behaviors that fuel the spread and growth of HIV/AIDS -- the race will beat the polar bear to extinction by about 50 years…

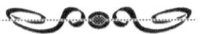

RISK FACTORS AMONG BLACKS & BARRIERS TO PREVENTION

Source References

- Anderson RN, Smith BL. Deaths: leading causes for 2001. *National Vital Statistics Reports* 2003;52(9): 27–33. Available at http://www.cdc.gov/nchs/data/nvsr/ nvsr52/nvsr52_09.pdf. Accessed December 23, 2004.
- CDC. *HIV/AIDS Surveillance Report, 2003* (Vol. 15). Atlanta: US Department of Health and Human Services, CDC; 2004:1–46. Available at http://www.cdc.gov/ hiv/stats/2003surveillancereport.pdf. Accessed February 2, 2005.
- CDC. Diagnoses of HIV/AIDS — 32 states, 2000–2003. *MMWR* 2004;53:1106–1110.
- CDC. Late versus early testing of HIV — 16 sites, United States, 2000–2003. *MMWR* 2003;52:581–586.
- Hader S, Smith D, Moore J, Holmberg S. HIV infection in women in the United States: status at the millennium. *JAMA* 2001;285:1186–1192.
- CDC. HIV transmission among black college student and non-student men who have sex with men — North Carolina, 2003. *MMWR* 2004;53:731–734.
- Montgomery JP, Mokotoff ED, Gentry AC, Blair JM. The extent of bisexual behaviour in HIV-infected men and implications for transmission to their female sex partners. *AIDS Care* 2003;15:829–837.
- Leigh B, Stall R. Substance use and risky sexual behavior for exposure to HIV: issues in methodology, interpretation, and prevention. *American Psychologist* 1993;48:1035–1045.
- Sharpe TT, Lee LM, Nakashima AK, Elam-Evans LD, Fleming P. Crack cocaine use and adherence to antiretroviral treatment among HIV-infected black women. *Journal of Community Health* 2004;29:117–127.
- (U.S. Dept. of Health and Human Services, *National Institute of Allergy and Infectious Diseases,* March 2005).
- CDC. *Sexually Transmitted Disease Surveillance, 2003*. Atlanta: US Department of Health and Human Services, CDC; September

2004. Available at http://www.cdc.gov/std/stats/toc2003.htm. Accessed February 2, 2005.

- Fleming DT, Wasserheit JN. From epidemiological synergy to public health policy and practice: the contribution of other sexually transmitted diseases to sexual transmission of HIV infection. *Sexually Transmitted Infections* 1999;75:3–17.
- CDC. HIV/AIDS among racial/ethnic minority men who have sex with men—United States, 1989–1998. *MMWR* 2000;49:4–11.
- CDC. HIV/STD risks in young men who have sex with men who do not disclose their sexual orientation—six US cities, 1994–2000. *MMWR* 2003;52:81–85.
- US Census Bureau. Poverty status of the population in 1999 by age, sex, and race and Hispanic origin. March 2000. Available at http://www.census.gov/prod/ 2003pubs/c2 kbr-19.pdf.   Accessed January 3, 2005.
- Diaz T, Chu S, Buehler J, et al. Socioeconomic differences among people with AIDS: results from a multistate surveillance project. *American Journal of Preventive Medicine* 1994;10:217–222.
- CDC. HIV transmission among black women—North Carolina, 2004. *MMWR* 2005;54:89–93.
- Trubo R. CDC initiative targets HIV research gaps in black and Hispanic communities. *JAMA* 2004;292: 2563–2564.
- HIV *Positive!*, June/July 2004

~~~~~~~~~~~~~~~~~~~

Medicinal Therapies

When HIV/AIDS first surfaced in the United States in 1981, there were no medicines to combat the disease and very few treatments existed for the opportunistic diseases that resulted. AIDS was a death sentence and there were no treatments available whatsoever. Scientists began to work feverishly to find a way to abate the spread of this new virus and its frightening ability to violently consume life. The first compound developed that proved to be effective was AZT (also known as Retrovir or Zidovudine). It is still a mainstay of HIV therapy even today, but was not very good by itself (HIV *Positive!*, June/July 2004).

During this period of slow drug-therapy development, it was common for people with HIV to swallow as many as 30 pills a day! In 1995/1996, however, scientists came up with the three-drug "cocktail", which turned HIV into a chronic, manageable disease (HIV *Positive!*, June/July 2004).

This, however, has proven to be a double-edged sword because while new drug therapies make living with HIV more of a reality than ever before, millions continue to die due to continual promiscuous, licentious behaviors. Some who are infected with HIV/AIDS think that having sex with an already-infected person will cause no further harm. This couldn't be further from the truth because *both parties* can develop a *new* form of AIDS that is completely non-responsive to existing drug therapies.

The U.S. Food and Drug Administration (FDA) has approved a number of drugs treating HIV infection, such as: AZT, ddC (zalcitabine), ddI (dideoxyinosine), d4T, abacavir (ziagen), and tenofovir (viread). These drugs may stop the spread of HIV in the body and delay the start of opportunistic infections. Other drugs that can be prescribed: non-nucleoside reverse transcriptase inhibitors (NNRTIs), such as, delvaridine (Rescriptor), Sustiva and nevirapine (Viramune), in combination with other antiretroviral drugs (United States Department of Health and Human Services, *National Institute of Allergy and Infectious Diseases,* March 2005).

More recently, the FDA has approved a second class of drugs to treat infection. These drugs, called "protease inhibitors," interrupt virus replication. They include: Ritonavir (Novir), Saquinivir (Invirase), Indinavir (Crixivan), Amprenivir (Agenerase), Nelfinavir (Viracept) and Lopinavir (Kaletra) United States Department of Health and Human Services, *National Institute of Allergy and Infectious Diseases,* March 2005.

Despite the beneficial effects of these drugs, however, HIV can become resistant to *any* of them. In this case, health care providers must use a combination treatment to effectively suppress the virus. When three or more inhibitors and protease inhibitors are used in combination, it is referred to as highly active antiretroviral therapy, or HAART, and can be used by people who are infected with HIV as well as people with AIDS (United States Department of Health and Human Services, *National Institute of Allergy and Infectious Diseases,* March 2005).

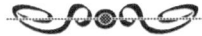

CHAPTER II

THE CLIMATE AND CULTURE

"It's yo' thang, do what you wanna do. I

cain't tell ya who to sock-it to…"

II. The Climate and Culture

Any meteorologist will make clear that the two key components needed to create the 'perfect storm' are timing and atmosphere. If the timing is right, the low pressure and high pressure systems meet and collide, you have it – the perfect storm. The *perfect* conditions existed in the climate of the 60s to brew up something of the nature and magnitude that it did. The two dynamics of time and atmosphere collided and produced devastating penalties, which have reverberated into this century and will beyond it.

As soon as Time's clock struck 12:00 a.m. the early morning of January 1, 1960, it appeared the total, natural world changed *inexplicably*, completely and forever. At the beginning of the decade, a radically bold change in attitudes became obvious and widespread – everywhere people were trumpeting 'Make Love, Not War' and violent rebellion became an ever-constant presence.

It was a wild, confusing, and for some, innocent era: 'free love,' war, flower children, *Buster Browns*, Leave It to Beaver, Vietnam, hippies, Eagle stamps, yippies, The Beatles, Cracker Jacks, Woodstock, riots, *Poll Parrott* sneakers, tie-dyed clothes, napalm, Andy Griffith, S&H green stamps, suicide, The Age of Aquarius and *Lucy in the Sky with Diamonds* (LSD). In response, the *world* was thrown off balance.

Who alive at the time is able to forget that torrid period? I'm sure if you were above the age of three you *can't* forget the 60s. The revolutions of that time were so powerful that the period dictates our existence even to this day. As I do, I'm sure you also refer back to that bittersweet period which was then a bewildered dream – but the *consequences* of that period have produced a nightmare. Vestiges of that period have bred cruel spawn...

The 1960s saw the beginning of a third kind of war. Up until then the world had been relatively calm and traditional on the social level. But now youngsters of the postwar generation were coming of age. Not liking the world they saw, and feeling its problems were being dealt with ineffectively, they embarked upon a war of their own—a war of protest. Demonstrations, riots and a general state of pandemonium defined the period. Social tension was so dense that it hung over the country like a soggy, wet blanket. *Everywhere* and with one voice people were demanding 'rights'.

Women wanted the 'right' to be treated as a man's equal in every arena – socially, politically, economically and sexually. Suddenly TV sitcoms like "Donna Reed" and "Leave It To Beaver", where Donna and June tipped around the house in 3-inch heels, wearing outfits fit for a runway, were no longer viewed as the model by which women wanted to pattern themselves. Women's perceived role as the menial, mild, subservient housekeeper and wearer-of-many-hats was unceremoniously chucked. Instead, she began boldly touting the popular commercial phrase, "I can bring home the bacon, fry it up in a pan and NEVER let you forget you're a man..." Demanding equality, women burned their bras, began popping the newly-introduced birth-control pill like M&Ms, left their domestic obligations of home in a miniskirt, high heels and a haircut, joined the workforce, created latch-key kids – and societal hell and havoc in her wake.

Men wanted the 'right' to refuse to go to war in a far country and dodge the draft without being carted off to prison. Negroes (which Blacks were called in the early 60s and in later 60s, African-Americans) wanted the 'right' to equality on *some* level of American society. Everyone was clamoring for 'rights' of some sort. But not only was this sentiment voiced in America -- the whole *world* chimed in...

Many a mile was walked in "ban the bomb" protests. In fact, almost anything that was deemed worthy of a protest warranted a march, a student strike, a sit-in, or an act of civil disobedience. Suddenly in youthful rebellion against authority, "Father Knows Best" became "Father Knows *Nothing.*" A majority of young people apparently supported this new kind of warfare, at least in principle. A poll of German youths taken in 1968 showed 67 percent in favor, leading the German newsmagazine *Der Spiegel* to comment: "When it comes to marching, most of them are willing to lend not only their hearts but also their feet and, if need be, their fists."

Author William Burroughs said in 1968: "The youth rebellion is a worldwide phenomenon that has not been seen before in history." In that year student unrest led to widespread riots and a general strike in France that almost brought down Charles de Gaulle's government. At the beginning of the decade, student protest actually had brought down a government, South Korea's, although at the cost of over 200 lives. And as regards protesting students in Japan, the book *1968 Weltpanorama* says: "Japan scarcely differs from America and Europe. At the most, Japanese students are only somewhat more imaginative than their fellow students in Berkeley, Paris, or Frankfurt."

Much of this protest was directed against war—war in general and the war in Vietnam in particular. At first the United States supplied the south with only military aid. But during the 1960s, it started sending troops, reaching a peak of over half a million before the decade was over. The war became like a festering sore that refused to heal. "In May 1965 a teach-in attended by twelve thousand students in the United States turned into an antiwar rally, and set the pattern for the massive campus antiwar demonstrations that marked the rest of the decade," says Charles R. Morris in his book '*A Time of Passion—America 1960-1980*'. To emphasize their stand, thousands of young men burned their draft cards. Some went even further, says Morris, giving two examples of men who "publicly burnt themselves to death to protest the war."

Many times while sitting in front of our 25-inch Zenith black and white TV console, eating lemon Jello or rice pudding after dinner, it was not uncommon to see pictures of the bloody Vietnam War. Soldiers with dirty faces and glazed eyes were peeking from foxholes, looking gaunt, afraid – and *young*. Historically, war and rebellion -- whether domestically or abroad -- has *always* precipitated major societal change. For one thing, there will always be those who feel why are we fighting for rights for some other country, when things are so *messed up* in our *own* backyard? Young people were dying then and young people are *yet* dying, fighting strange wars in strange lands. What is there *left* to have freedom or rights to?

While many were fighting and dying in Vietnam in the 60s, some of us were fighting and dying right here in America. We watched the racist sheriff in the South, Bull Connor, as he turned the powerful, watery-fury of fire hoses and unleashed vicious dogs on terrified blacks (many of whom were women and children) as they demonstrated for the civil rights of equality and social freedom. I watched Gov. George Wallace as he *himself* blocked entrance to the school to prevent black students from attending. I witnessed the sit-ins of the South, of the North and heard about Jim Clark, George Wallace and "Bloody Sunday" in Selma, Alabama. Even now I remember the tragedy of the deaths of the four young girls in the Alabama church bombing in 1964, the deaths of the three young men Chaney, Schwerner and Goodman who were killed during a voter registration drive and their bodies were later found in a dam.

I can recall in St. Louis during the early 60s my mother taking all of her seven children to the Woolworth's store on Grand. We would each order a hamburger with fries, once a month. People would look at all of us and sometimes smile. But others *didn't* – like the woman who took Mama's order. When I think about it now, I don't ever remember sitting at the lunch counter of Woolworth's…

On Hamilton street (*1418*, to be exact…), we had white neighbors who were very friendly: Tom & Mary Lou, who lived next door, were married and had a daughter named Lynn. At the age of six, I received my first formal birthday present -- from Lynn. It was a large coloring book with more crayons than I'd ever seen in one box, all wrapped in beautiful, colorful paper. Even though Mama always baked each of us a huge cake of our choice for birthdays, I can remember even now how excited I was over Lynn's gift. I'll never forget it…

We had other white neighbors: the interesting, eccentric Mr. Erskine from Scotland smoked a pipe and sometimes wore a kilt! The only thing missing were the bagpipes… At least once a month, he gave my family some wonderful cinnamon bread. And the Sullivans, who lived at the corner, could always be found either gardening in the back or reading the newspaper on the front porch. The Hollidays around the corner had a small store in their basement, and turned out the best hamburgers in the *world*! *Every cent* my siblings and I could rake or scrape up went to purchase one of those fantastic burgers and a bag of chips…

It was a wonderful, *peaceful* time in my memory -- when 'new technology' was limited to Mama getting a Princess-style phone in place of the heavy black phone with the rotary dial. But it all changed suddenly, drastically and irrevocably. Around 1963, there was a noticeable shift in the neighborhood – 'white flight' and urban blight began setting in. During this tense time, something horrible happened to the nice Sullivans at the end of the block, which precipitated white flight from our neighborhood. It was said that three black youth caught Mr. Sullivan as he was gardening in his backyard, and beat him so badly he had to be hospitalized. When Mrs. Sullivan tried to stop them, she was also beaten. Mr. Sullivan eventually died from the injuries he received. To this day, however, we never heard what happened to Mrs. Sullivan after that terrible incident...

One by one, the once proud Wellston shopping district which boasted stores like J.C. Penney, and which was back in the day the equivalent to a Macy's, disappeared almost overnight. The wonderful Wellston library where Betty got her first job, closed up. The upscale Albert's shoe store where Andrew worked, the elegant Cunningham's and Gardner's stores where Mama bought her beautiful Sunday clothes and hats when our family 'had money,' the Fox Camera and Record store, all *closed*. Woolworth's closed up; so did Three Sisters and The Libson Shop. Pretty soon, Wellston resembled a ghost town, with only a Jupiter store and Central Hardware remaining at the further end. For well over 30 years Wellston lay abandoned and in ruins, and even today with the *turtle*-slow 'urban renewal' that is alleged to soon take place, it will be but a *shadow* of its former self.

So *much* was going on around 1963: Medgar Evers and Malcolm X were assassinated, the race riots in Detroit and California started. I remember watching over and over again the assassination of President John F. Kennedy and the long, drawn, *hopeless* faces of weary people crying – mine being one of them...

Who can forget the charismatic Dr. Martin Luther King's electrifying "I Have A Dream" speech during the *March on Washington* on August 28, 1963, in which 250,000 showed up? As Dr. King preached his message of God-given human rights in response to racial brutality, my mother yelled in the background that he was going to 'get hisself killed!' And he *did* – one sad day in April... Just recently the world lost two of the last, great icons of the Civil Rights era: Rosa Parks and Coretta Scott King. Whatever will we do without their humanity?

Has anything changed since that morally deprived and depraved, racially biased, angst-riddled period? Not really. In 1963 during a television interview the intense author, James Baldwin, stated: "I am terrified of the moral apathy – the death of the heart which is happening in my country. How, precisely, are you going to reconcile yourself to your situation here and how are you going to communicate to the vast, heedless, unthinking, cruel …. majority that you *are* here -- and to be *here* means that you cannot be anywhere else?" Nearly 50 years later, a certain ethnic group is *yet* attempting to define, justify and reconcile its role and presence in this country.

Attitudes of this age echo the credo established during the 60s time period. The selfish mindset of "anything goes" and determined rebellion against conventional, true and *God*-ordained principles remains as the social, cultural, political and spiritual countenance of the world. On the following pages are listed several sources that continue to greatly impact our culture, especially our children, and has contributed significantly to the ever-accelerating downward spiral of society, producing 30-year old grandmothers, 10-year old alcoholics and 5-year old murderers…

1. Television

By definition, the media is an agent or means of propagating information or ideas (e.g., radio, TV, movies, magazines, billboards, etc.) The media has historically played an important role in advancing certain lifestyles and ideas. Some important, landmark media events have contributed to the shift in sexual views and attitudes, beginning in the 1920s (the introduction of nude calendars, the first *Playboy* magazine was published in 1953, etc.) that fanned the flames of a rapidly growing culture of promiscuous sexuality in America.

Children today watch an incredible amount of television. The average child spends 1,154 hours watching TV and only 900 hours in school per year. Even *cartoons* nowadays need to be adult-rated: The Family Guy, American Hero, South Central, etc.

- The average American teenager will view nearly 14,000 sexual references, innuendoes and jokes per year
- A child has seen 200,000 violent acts and 16,000 murders on television by age 18
- MTV broadcasts an average of 18 physical and 17 verbal references to sex *per hour*
- Studies have found that teens who watch a lot of television with sexual content are *twice* as likely to engage in sexual intercourse as those who watch fewer such programs

- A study of 1,792 adolescents ages 12-17 showed that watching sex on TV influences teens to have sex. Youths who watched more sexual content were more likely to initiate intercourse and progress to more advanced non-coital sexual activities in the year following the beginning of the study. Youths in the 90th percentile of TV sex viewing had a predicted probability of intercourse initiation that was approximately double that of youths in the 10th percentile. Basically, kids with higher exposure to sex on TV were almost twice as likely to initiate sexual intercourse, than kids with lower exposure.

- In a sample of programming from the 2001-2002 TV season, sexual content appeared in 64% of all TV programs. Those programs with sexually related material had an average of 4.4 scenes per hour.

Talk of sex is more frequent (61%) vs. overt portrayals (32%). One out of every 7 programs includes a portrayal of sexual intercourse.

- Portrayals that included sexual risks (STDS or becoming pregnant), abstinence or need for sexual safety was depicted in 15% of the shows with sexual content. Hence, sexual content on TV is more likely to *promote* sexual activity among US adolescents than it is to discourage it.

- Factors positively associated with initiation of intercourse among virgins are: Watching sex on TV, having older friends, getting low grades, engaging in deviant behavior. Positive factors for virgins to abstain are: parental monitoring, parent education, living with both parents, having parents who would disprove of adolescent sex, being religious, and having good mental health.

Suggested guidelines...

- While the media can be held partly responsible for the effects their shows have on their audiences, parents have the power – and the *responsibility* -- to control the influences children face. Help your children monitor the amount of TV they watch, and even more importantly, *what* they watch.
- Consider canceling your cable subscription. Cable TV offers many inappropriate channels. By receiving only the local channels, your teens won't have the temptation to watch as much TV, and are less likely to be exposed to perverse materials. The sacrifice is well worth it!
- Only allow your teen to watch a certain number of hours of TV per week and encourage them to do something stimulating with their time
- Watch TV with your children and *speak up* when there is improper content. *Lead by example* and turn off the TV when inappropriate sexual scenes are shown. *Be the parent!*
- Bring your family together *by keeping the TV off* during mealtimes and family discussions. You will be surprised how this seemingly small thing will improve your family's relationship!

Common Sense Media
www.commonsensemedia.org

Parent's Television Council
www.parentstv.org

2. Video Games

In the Super Mario Brothers game of the 80s, players pounced on bad guys' heads and search for gold coins. However, in 2004's top-selling video game, *Grand Theft Auto*, players slit cops' throats and prowl for prostitutes.

Video games can be even worse than passive entertainment like TV and movies, because instead of just *observing* violence and immorality, players are now able – via the rapid advances of modern technology – to actively participate in killing, drug dealing and even sex. In fact, 48% of video game content involving violence, sexual themes, profanity, substance abuse, and/or gambling, is not even labeled on the game's box. An alarming 14% of 8th and 9th grade video gamers are considered "addicted" to this activity.

With the ability to interact with the video games, children can use "virtual" banks, policemen, women, etc. to plan and practice their deadly tirades. As has been proven time and again, television and video games can lead to imitation. With ever-increasing violence and gore, video games have been named as the root cause of many of today's tragedies in schools: the Columbine murders were directly linked to the video game "Doom".

A recent episode of *CSI: Miami* (November 21, 2005) dealt with "a new kind of criminal", as Horatio put it. Five teenaged boys went into a bank, shot out the cameras, killed a teller, took money and attempted to rape another teller. One robber was killed in the process. They wore hideous masks and later the money was found, which had been *dumped* by the felons. Apparently, the entire robbery had been based on a video game and for every action the boys took, there was a point value associated with it. They killed and robbed simply for the thrill of it and the accumulation of points in a game.

These games are not movies, nor are they spectator games. Rather, they are realistic simulations that can train a child to drive – *or kill…* The games use techniques known to be effective in teaching young people. *Simulation* is designed to polish the trainee's instincts, to help them build habits that they can carry out quickly, without second thoughts. Video games laced with human slaughter desensitizes and helps young, impressionable people practice killing.

In his book *The Deathmatch Manifesto,* Robert Waring analyzes the popularity of so-called deathmatch games among adolescents. Mr. Waring believes that an underground society of gamers has sprung up around this phenomenon. These games really have the effect, not of educating, but of teaching to kill. Adolescents are intrigued by the force of the three-dimensional scenarios designed as backdrops for the bloody struggles. "Playing with a live opponent from anywhere in the world, and trying to prove yourself, is a powerful experience. It's really easy to get sucked into that," Waring comments.

Not having access through the Internet, some buy video-game packages to use on the television at home. Others customarily go to public places where they rent video-game machines and have 'virtual' fights to the death with other opponents.

Over 1,000 studies - including a Surgeon General's special report in 1972 and a National Institute of Mental Health report 10 years later - attest to a causal connection between media violence and aggressive behavior in some children. Studies show that the more "real-life" the violence portrayed, the greater the likelihood that it will be "learned." **American Academy of Pediatrics Policy Statement, Volume 95, Number 6 - June 1995**

Media violence may cause aggressive and antisocial behavior, desensitize viewers to future violence and increase perceptions that they are living "in a mean and dangerous world." **- American Academy of Pediatrics**

"A steady diet of violent content over time creates a culture that tells kids that violence is the accepted way we solve our problems." **- Ibid - Attributed to Kathryn C. Montgomery, President of the Center for Media Education.**

The cumulative impact of violence-laden imagery can lead to a "mean-world" perspective, in which viewers have an unrealistically dark view of life. **- The Christian Science Monitor, November 18, 1996**

Suggested Guidelines…

- Be aware of the types of games your teen plays, or at least watch them while they play. If for some reason they object or start to feel uncomfortable with you viewing and/or participating, it may be a sign that they shouldn't be playing the game in the first place.
- Be sure to voice your concerns regarding any inappropriate content.
- Video games have the tendency to consume many hours of young people's lives. Consider setting a time limit for how long your youth are allowed to play.

Here's Help!

Focus on the Family
www.pluggedonline.com

Game Spot
www.gamespot.com/misc/top100_pop.html

Fun Home Games
www.funhomegames.com

3. Sex/Dating

The term 'sex' can mean many things to many people. Among youths it can refer to private masturbation, oral sex, group sex and intercourse. Teens also seem inclined to have multiple sex partners. Various studies show that 1 in 5 high school students will have four or more sex partners in their lifetime, 1 in 10 will have seven or more partners, and 1 in 3 females and 1 in 2 males will have six or more partners by the time they reach 21.

One study of young women between the ages of 12 and 18, who had their first sexual experience prior to age 15 revealed the primary reasons for their decision to have sex was they were 'pressured' into it by an older partner (usually rape or molestation), friends were 'doing it', they were curious and they wanted to feel grown up. The book *Young Unwed Fathers* observes: "To many boys [in the inner city], sex is an important symbol of local social status; sexual conquests become so many notches on one's belt. Many of the girls offer sex as a gift in their bargaining for the attentions of a young man."

As we have seen, sexual intercourse without moral restraints can be devastating socially, personally and medically. The pressure to be sexually active is very real in a teenager's life. In fact, **46%** of high school students in the United States have had sexual intercourse. **40%** of 10th graders engaged in oral sex in the past year, with a quarter of them reporting three or more partners. According to one survey, 14% of 13 and 14 years say they are sexually active, meaning they have gone beyond kissing. That number jumps to 41% when kids reach 15 and 16. One case of an STD is diagnosed for every 4 sexually active teens.

According to a report in the *American Journal of Public Health*, a study done by University of Albany's School of Criminal Justice found a direct relationship between childhood sexual abuse and teen prostitution. The report indicated that early childhood abuse and/or neglect was a significant predictor of prostitution. Females who were sexually abused were three times more likely to end up in teenage prostitution than those not abused.

Although sex is common, most sexually active teens wish they had waited longer to have sex, which suggest that sex is occurring before youths are prepared for its consequences. A study done by the *Journal of Adolescent Health,* however, shows a direct link between parent-child relationships as playing a significant role in teen sexuality. It was discovered that teens that didn't feel close to their mothers or fathers had sex by the time they turned 17 years old. However, teens that *were* satisfied with their relationship with their parents were 3 times less likely to engage in sex. Unhealthy parent-child relationships can result in teens making sexually unwise choices.

Many young people use sex to verify their attractiveness and desirability. In the current culture of materialism and physical beauty, this once-considered naive act of adolescence is causing a great many young, premature deaths. Many youngsters are frankly unaware of the consequences of sex in this disease-ravaged age. But high-risk sexual behavior does not have to be the norm for adolescents. Like drug use, most sexual behaviors are a choice. One thing is certain: *no one has ever caught AIDS from being abstinent.* You have the power to *choose* not to have sex at all, or if you've been sexually active in the past, you can *choose to stop.* It can be high risk or *no* risk. *You have the power to decide your own fate and destiny.* It's all up to you...

Suggested Guidelines

- Don't be afraid to ask the hard questions and to openly discuss sex with your youth.
- Children are eager to grow up too fast. Depending on your child's maturity level, discuss an appropriate age for them to begin looking for date-worthy relationships.
- Encourage your youth to bring their "significant other" to your house so you can meet them and spend time getting to know them (and get a "feel" of what the relationship is like).
- Teach your kids to be self-confident and their *own person.* Many lives have been ruined because they weren't strong enough to say "no".
- Teach your kids to make wise decisions in their relationships with the opposite sex, such as never being alone in a bedroom and never

being alone in the house. It would also save you a lot of headaches if you set a curfew.

- Encourage your teen to set solid physical boundaries in their relationships.

Here's Help!

Joshua Harris, *"I Kissed Dating Good-Bye & Boy Meets Girl"*
Dannah Gresh, *"The Bride Wore White: Seven Secrets to Sexual Purity"*

4. Friends

One of the biggest reasons young people make wrong choices is because of friends and other close associations. The most effective, influential peer pressure often comes from these associations.

Many of today's young people are getting pressured from all sides: family, school, and society at large to 'do better', 'make me proud,' 'make the grade' and 'fit in'. Even the *thought* of it is overwhelming. Small wonder why young people feel they have to 'keep up' appearances. This results in the wearing of many masks by our children – and it is difficult to perceive what they are really thinking or feeling.

It can be a very lonely life when young people feel they are the only ones trying to 'do the right thing' – and other young people can be cruel. The daily news is riddled with stories about how violent crimes are being committed -- by seemingly younger and younger people all the time -- after being bullied, pressured, dared and double-dared.

Who can forget the two friends, Eric Harris and Dylan Klebold, who orchestrated the 'Littleton Massacre' at Columbine high school, which resulted in the worst display of school violence in history, with the tragic loss of life of 15. It was stated that "the hardest thing about the search for an explanation was the growing fear there might not be one."

Dylan Klebold was said to be the weaker spirit of the two: quiet, reserved, looking for a leader, which he found in Eric Harris. It was said that on the day before the shooting, neighbors of the Harrises saw Klebold's black BMW parked outside Eric's house. Parents of neither of the youths had the vaguest idea of what was transpiring in their own home, with their own child – right under their nose. Parents, it is crucial to the physical, spiritual, emotional and mental development of your child that you know their closest friends and associates, and ensure they are respectable.

- It is almost impossible to know at all times who your child's friends or acquaintances are. So do the next best thing: get your child to talk about them by asking their names, what they are like, etc.
- Get to know the people your youth is hanging out with! This cannot be stressed enough. Do not be afraid to voice your concerns!
- Teens often feel like they're the only one trying to do right, but that's never completely true. Help your teen grow in their faith in God by getting them involved in a solid church youth group.
- If your teen is hanging out with the wrong crowd, point out specific ways you've noticed the change in them. Hopefully, this may help them take a second look at their friendships – and themselves…

5. Music

In the late 1960s and early 1970s, there was a dramatic, discernible shift in the medium of music. Lyrics became more sexually explicit, and nothing was left to the imagination. However, just in the last decade alone, we have experienced an even more remarkable decline in morality of the music industry, with the introduction of music videos.

With today's "music" saturated with vile sexual connotations – filled with f-, m-, b- and s- words that slander women, ethnic groups, Christianity -- up to and including encouraging murder and suicide -- something needs to be done to ban the distribution and sell of this type of material. In France, for example, rappers advocated the killing of police and police were killed by some who heard the music.

Youth today listen to the lyrics in this popular music – even when they *say* they aren't. Teens claim that they don't listen to the words but if you put them to the test, they can easily sing along. With radios blasting so loudly that they shake the very ground, youth *listen* and *absorb*. It is a known fact that many youth often go to bed with headphones on and whatever they happen to be listening to is *internalized*. Subliminal suggestion is entirely possible. You *do not* want your child internalizing evil! It will have a lifelong negative impact upon their life.

Suggested Guidelines

- With all the sex, violence and lies embedded in secular music, it would be a wise decision to not let your teens listen to secular music at all
- *Know what your child is listening to!* It is a good idea that parents know what's going on in their children's world and *become involved.* Even though this may make you uncomfortable, *learn the language*, music and everything else that applies to developing your child's character. Grab your youth's favorite CD cover and read the lyrics. What you find may surprise you – and can be an essential learning tool of your child and his times.
- *Do not allow your youth to listen at all to music that is too objectionable even for you!*

Here's Help!

Fresh Releases
www.freshreleases.com/rock.htm

Grading the Movies
www.gradingthemovies.com

6. Internet

The internet can be a wonderful tool – the world's biggest library. Magazines, newspapers, photographs and recordings on virtually every subject are at your fingertips. It can allow you to travel to distant lands – without leaving your living room. Little wonder, then, that experts say that over **350 million accessed the internet** last year!

With schools and libraries promoting internet use, millions of young people have access to it. In the United States alone, nearly 65 percent of youths between the ages of 12 and 19 have already used or subscribed to on-line services. Many use it for schoolwork. *BUT...*

It can happen quite by accident – the first time anyway. A pop-up just came out of *nowhere* – and curiosity killed the cat! **Ninety percent (90%) of 8-16 year olds have viewed porn online**, most of them while innocently doing homework. In fact, the average age of first exposure to internet porn is 11 years old, which has led to 12-17 year olds becoming its largest consumers. Pornography distorts young minds with unrealistic and temptation-laden imagery and it has ripped apart countless marriages and families.

But pornography isn't the Internet's *only* danger. **Eighty-nine percent of sexual solicitations of youth are made in chat rooms**. How many times have the headlines screamed of a young innocent falling prey to a sexual predator, whom they met in a *chat room*? Writer Leah Rozen observed: "Techno-savvy teenagers are spending hours chatting online with anonymous strangers all over the country and, even, the world. Unfortunately, some of those strangers with whom teens may be talking online also happen to be adult perverts looking for sexual trysts with kids." An article in *Popular Mechanics* warned that "you have to be extremely careful" when using public chat rooms. Giving out your name or address to a stranger could be an invitation to serious trouble.

An amazing **one-third** of adult internet users in the United States have visited some type of sexual site, a recent survey on on-line sex revealed. Vast numbers of people are now giving in to their sexual urges through the internet. "This is a hidden public health hazard exploding, in part, because very few are recognizing it *as such* or taking it seriously," says Dr. Al Cooper, the psychologist who conducted the survey.

Who are especially vulnerable to such cybersex? "Those users whose sexuality may have been suppressed and limited all their lives" but who "suddenly find an infinite supply of sexual opportunities" on the Internet, says Dr. Cooper. Most of those who frequent sexual sites, however, consider the practice to be harmless. But just as a drug addict develops a tolerance for the drug on which he is hooked, many cybersex addicts seek an increased "dose" of sexuality on the internet to gratify their cravings. They may even jeopardize their job and their relationship with their companion.

Researchers have found that "at least 200,000 Internet users are hooked on pornography sites, X-rated chat rooms or other sexual materials online," reports *The New York Times*. The study was conducted by psychologists at Stanford and Duquesne universities and is one of the first to have estimated the number of Internet "cybersex compulsives." The researchers said that these individuals visit X-rated Web sites more than 11 hours a week.

Sadly, many of cyberporn's viewers are children. Youngsters who are prohibited by law from purchasing pornographic literature or from renting pornographic videos can gain access to these in their own home with a few clicks of the mouse. The choices are endless. Many children regularly visit Internet sites without their parents' knowledge. In fact, *The Detroit News* states that "more than two in five children have subscribed to a web site or other service online even though nearly 85 percent of parents have rules against doing so."

While most children—and adults as well—are careful to hide the fact that they dabble in pornography, not everyone sees the need to do so. Some consider the practice to be a harmless form of recreation. Others concede that pornography is not good for children but reason that what adults do in private is their own business...

Suggested Guidelines

- To discourage the possibility of your youth viewing objectionable content on your computer, keep it in a public room where others can see the monitor at all times.
- In today's vein of parents wanting their children "to have more than I did", we have let our children down and exposed them to much more danger because of our refusal to "invade their privacy" and closely scrutinize their activity. Many parents have placed computers in their children's room and allowed them to place a "Private" sign on the door to keep parents out. Do you know what

you are encouraging? Not only is the child not being supervised, but they also get the impression that they can do whatever they want because "my parents don't care…" Once again, *you're* the parent, so don't be afraid to enforce rules!

- Late night surfing is often when temptation strikes. Have a "no Internet" rule after most of the family has gone to bed.
- *Make sure your teen knows to never give out any personal information in a chat room!* It's best to simply avoid them at all cost.
- To cut down on the possibility that your child may access porn or something objectionable on your computer, *allow them to only use the internet at the local library.* In this way, you can rest assured they will not have access to objectionable material due to safeguards.

Here's Help!

Covenant Eyes Internet Accountability
www.convenanteyes.com

7. Movies

Variety magazine reports that films featuring graphic violence and sex are on the increase, while wholesome, family films are hardly being made at all. "Sex sells," and Hollywood monopolizes on it. More and more promiscuity, violence and profanity are filling our theaters and our homes, all in the name of "entertainment." Is this having an effect on the young, impressionable youth who watch it? Yes, it is!

"Hedonism, sexuality, violence, greed, selfishness", according to child psychiatrist Robert Coles, are the values dominating in most movies being produced today. Research organized by Dr. Vince Hammond likewise concluded that "most of the films shown in the industrialized countries contained at least some violence, with many being rated violent or highly violent." Hammond's researchers surveyed 1,000 films from a variety of countries. "The production of violent films is a *global* problem."

Recently, movies that have been rated PG-13 would have received nothing less than "R" in years past, for content like nudity, sexual scenes, language, and drug and alcohol depictions. Junior high students who watched multiple movies that depicted alcohol usage were three times more likely to try drinking than those who don't. It also works the same for movies laden with violence, drug use, vulgarity and sex. Movies mount a powerful assault on the senses. When you focus on the larger-than-life images that move across the big screen, you can virtually surrender your mind to the will of the moviemaker...

Suggested Guidelines

- Set standards and guidelines as to what kind of movies your family will watch. For example, you can decide as a family not to watch R-rated movies or movies with sexual themes.
- Do you know what kind of movies your children are watching? Make it a point to.

Here's Help!

Grading the Movies
www.gradingthemovies.com

8. Drugs/Alcohol

Drug and alcohol abuse are at the top of the list as being the most risk-taking and self-destructive behaviors of young people. By a matter of degrees, youths push the envelope to ever-accelerating destructive behavior. The reason many become addicted is their bad association with those who are abusing alcohol and drugs. Peer pressure and curiosity often play a significant role to the path of drug and alcohol abuse for these youth. A U.S. survey revealed that a shocking **41 percent** of high school seniors go on an alcohol binge *every two weeks*!

A recent study shows that 47.1% of high schoolers have abused alcohol, and 23.9% have used marijuana in the past 30 days! 28.5% say drugs were offered to them on school premises. Studies have shown that if you start drinking at the age of 15, you have a 28% chance of eventually becoming an alcoholic. This is especially troubling when the average age of a first-time drinker is **12**... However, it is not uncommon to hear of children as young as *eight* finding their way into the family's wine cabinet and drinking.

The pressure to be socially accepted is one of the major reasons young people indulge in drinking and drugs. Other reasons include an unhealthy home environment, boredom, curiosity, anger, immaturity, thrill seeking, denial of the dangers, the desire to look 'cool', low self-confidence, low self-worth and to reduce stress.

One assumption made by youth -- and adults as well -- who try drugs and/or alcohol is '*I can handle it*'. This is a fallacy. People who become involved lose control of their abilities to think straight and make balanced decisions, causing undesired consequences. Sometimes it's not the substance itself that kills or maims – it's the action a person takes while under the influence that causes serious harm. For instance, driving while under the influence in alcohol-related accidents kills someone every thirty minutes and injures another person every two minutes in the United States.

I know firsthand of the devastation that is caused to the family of victims killed by drunk or drug-impaired drivers. My lovely 11-year old niece, Esther Ruth, was killed in May 2006 by a drunk driver. There is no reason that can be offered to justify using a car as a *murder weapon* – destroying such a precious, vital life...

A study of male adolescent addicts revealed that more than a third had been physically abused. Another study of 178 adult alcoholic women found that 88 percent had been severely mistreated in one way or another.

The book *Addictions* explains: "The classic path for addicts is that, somewhere along the line, they start to hate themselves, and they become hideously tormented by the hold their addiction has gained." Many who are dependent on alcohol or drugs use them as escape routes from emotional crises. According to the *American Psychiatric Association*, a person is probably addicted to a substance if:

- The substance is taken in larger amounts

- Attempts have been unsuccessful to 'cut down' on the use of the substance, and you experience withdrawal when attempting to stop

- Things that were once important (job, sports, etc.) are discontinued
- More of the substance is needed to get the desired effects

Street Names for MARIJUANA/HASHISH – can be smoked ('blunts'), mixed with food or brewed

Grass, pot, herb, joints, Mary Jane, reefer, ganja, skunk, sinsemilla. For hashish – boom, chronic, gangster, hash, hash brownie, hash oil, hemp, Bubble Gum, Juicy Fruit, Northern Lights

Effects: Gives feeling of euphoria, causes confusion, impairs balance, causes paranoia, slows thinking and ability to react

Health Risks: Causes frequent respiratory infections, panic attacks, impaired memory, increases heart rate, anxiety

Street Names for INHALANTS – chemicals found in common household cleaners (spray paint, deodorant, paint thinner, nail polish and remover, felt-tip markers, rubber cement, super glue, dry-cleaning fluid, whipped-cream aerosols). Can be 'huffed', inhaled from soaked rags, containers, or substance-filled bags, sniffed from shirt cuffs or sleeves, inhaled from balloons

Amys, bang, head cleaner, kick, huff, moon gas, rush, whippets, poor man's pot, pearls

Effects: Gives short-lasting high, reduces inhibitions, causes headaches, slurred speech and loss of equilibrium

Health Risks: Can cause unconsciousness, can be immediately addicting, damages the cardiovascular system, nervous system and can cause sudden death

Street Names for ECTASY – tablets (various colors) imprinted with cartoon characters, commercial logos, smiley faces, clover leaves

Ectasy, Adam, Eve, XTC, X, peace, STP, essence, love drug, hug drug, Scooby snacks, speed for lovers, B-bombs, E, sweeties

Effects: Increases sensory abilities: love, compassion, empathy. Feelings of euphoria, increases mental alertness, rapid heart or irregular heartbeat, causes weight loss, nervousness, insomnia, paranoia, chills, involuntary teeth grinding, blurred vision

Health Risks: Can cause immediate addiction, depression, impaired learning abilities, cardiac damage, very high fever, liver and kidney failure, and irreversible damage to brain cells

Suggested Guidelines

- Teenagers often drink/do drugs in order to meet a need for identity, acceptance or belonging. It is important that teens have *their own* personal reasons for not doing drugs, alcohol or *sex* – which generally comes into the picture with the other two addictions.
- Be sure to talk with your children about the 'why nots' of these dangerous abuses.
- Teenage years are perhaps the most difficult time in anyone's life. It is important that your children know that you are there for them. Let them know that you love and accept them, but even better yet, God loves and accepts them for who He made them to be.

Here's Help!

Educating Voices
www.educatingvoices.org

The Partnership for a Drug-Free America
www.drugfree.org

9. Too Much…

Today's youth are overwhelmed with activity. There's school, sports practice and events, after school jobs, band practice, and hours of homework – not to mention the Friday night choir rehearsal or usher board meeting… Teens are constantly on the run -- going, going, going. Many teens are so heavily involved in various activities that they become stressed and turn to various unsavory alternatives (drugs, sex, alcohol, etc.) in an attempt to keep up with the demand.

True, an idle mind is the devil's workshop. However, too much of *any* thing is still too much (even *church*…). Involvement is good but involvement to the point of exhaustion and taxation does much more harm than good in the long run. It is quite easy to become burned-out on practically *anything* that is done ritualistically, or according to a set schedule. Strangely, routine has a way of causing disorientation.

Suggested Guidelines

- Teach your teens that God comes first and when they are on their own, they will follow your example
- Teach your children how to acquire and maintain a healthy *balance* in life. Teach them the importance of work -- and rest.

Here's Help!

Global Expeditions Mission Trips
www.globalexpeditions.com

THE CLIMATE AND CULTURE

Source References

- Watch Tower Bible and Tract Society, *"1960-1969: The 1960's—A Period of Turbulent Protest"*, 1987
- The Fact Index, *"The 1960s"*
- BattleCry For a Generation, *"Youth Culture Crisis Guide"*, 2005
- Dr. Dale Conaway, *"Sex & The Bible"*, Destiny Image Publishers, Inc.
- TIME Magazine, "The Year In Medicine From A to Z", December 2004
- TV Turnoff, *"Images, Facts and Figures"* Fact Sheet
- Studies Conducted by *RAND* and published in the September 2004 issue of *Pediatrics*.
- Watch Tower Bible and Tract Society, *"Death in Video Games and on the Internet"*, July 2000
- The Washington Herald, *"Violent Video Games are Training Children to Kill"*
- Watchtower Bible and Tract Society, *"Fathers – Why They Are Disappearing?"*, 2000
- TIME Magazine, *"Special Report: The Littleton Massacre,"* May 3, 1999
- Watchtower Bible and Tract Society, *"Freedom of Speech in the Home: Is It A Ticking Time Bomb?"* July 1996
- Ibid, *"How Can I Avoid Dangers on the Internet?"* January 2000
- Ibid, *"Does It Matter Which Movies I See?"* July 2002
- Ibid, *"Who Gets Hooked and Why?"* April 1994
- Joan Esherick, *"The Silent Cry"*, Mason Crest Publishers

CHAPTER III

THE CONSEQUENCE

"When the end of the world finally happens, we shouldn't be surprised. It's been comin' for a long time, man..."

- Marilyn Manson

III. The Consequence: AIDS

The pursuit of happiness and fulfillment through self-gratification has produced nothing but frustration, emptiness, disease – and death. Our societal structure has been weakened on every level of civilization. A society without standards is a *weak*, crumbling society – a victim of tragic history by its own hand.

Across the board the essential, defining element of love is nonexistent and has been replaced by the egocentric behaviors of lust, greed and avarice, producing addictions of all sorts. Even the decent, moral traits of compassion and concern have been traded for apathy and coldness. Lust is the implicit order of the time – lust for power, money, our pound of flesh, me, my, mine, I – forsaking, neglecting, forgetting, abandoning, misusing, abusing all others… Clearly, an acquired deficiency in *love* is prevalent in all areas of humanity: for family, for God, for self, for others. Hence, the reason:

- In Family, a husband can tell his wife 'I've outgrown you' and she responds 'you're not the same person I married', and this justifies divorce and the ruination of *many* lives. The absence of love in family is the reason for affairs of all kinds. It's why men go on the down-low and why women go on the up and up, while another man is coming up from the down low…
- In Church, the absence of love is depicted in the 'religious' who can cluck their tongues and shake their heads in judgment of a city bared by a fierce wind, in which Satan was riding, going 'to and fro in the earth' seeking whom he could destroy (Job 2:2, I Peter 5:8). Many were *deceived* in thinking that God who is *just* would spare St. Louis, California, Florida, or New York sinners yet wipe out New Orleans, Mississippi and Texas sinners.
- An absence of love is apparent in mordant seers who make glib references to the 'judgment' of God, *blaspheming* His name and character as they proclaim that *the* God of Love was responsible for killing *babies*, while allowing Bourbon Street in the French Quarter -- where half a world has *wallowed* in debauchery -- to remain virtually unscathed and in business throughout the entire devastation of a city…

- In Politics, an absence of love is palpable in politicians who bray that they are 'pro-life', yet wield a pen signing laws into policy that eradicate and annihilate lives, just as assuredly as if the pen were a sword. They assert that they are pro-life, yet without hesitation, send our young men and women to fight and die in strange lands – and for *what*? While piously declaring pro-life sentiments, they cut Medicare and Medicaid to the bare bone, making it necessary for the elderly to choose between either food or medicine, though they need *both* to live…

- An absence of love and truth is portrayed in a country that stamps 'In God We Trust' on every form of its currency, yet deny God's existence by acquiescing to every strident plea of atheists who claim infringement upon their rights. Yet have no problem violating *my* religious rights by banning prayer from schools, and by removing any *vestige* of God

- There is a blatant absence of love when a country can hypocritically respond to a disaster most of a world away within a day, dropping food and supplies from planes in parts of that country that had never seen human habitation. Yet when the worst disaster of our time transpired on *this* soil, it took nearly *a week* for troops to arrive, just so they could ignore, pass up and bark orders at the nearly-dead, and 'supervise' the distribution of water and packaged food -- armed with weaponry as though they were fighting a war in Iraq…

- In Society, something is clearly wrong and the absence of love for others is obvious when a homeless or abused *dog* warrants a spot on the evening news, and there is such a massive outpouring of love and concern for this *dog*. Yet, when a *human being* is homeless he will *remain* homeless if there is no shelter space available. No phones are ringing off the hook for the *human* homeless and it *certainly* won't make the evening news…

- The absence of love for self and their people is unfortunately displayed in an entire race of people, plunging helter-skelter towards extinction -- knowingly and willingly -- appeasing the very lusts that will bring about their end…

~~~~~~~~~~~~~~~~

Millions of young people today are tasting the bitterness of society's 'sour grapes'—paying the brutal penalty for its foolish and reckless sins of the past. Particularly distressing is the fact that the legacy is often passed on from generation to generation—a continuing cycle of pain and misery. The research is simply overwhelming in demonstrating that children are exposed to a plethora of physical, emotional, mental and spiritual deficiencies as a result.

This era of youth has experienced the worst breakdown of family in history, not only born into dysfunctional homes but also unnoticed by dysfunctional churches. It has experienced the ill-fated results of failed governmental systems and insufficient social programs, because the spiritual and moral element has been negated.

It is not uncommon today to find a 30-year old grandmother -- *babies* having babies. Few youths have either the emotional maturity or the experience to handle the demands of parenthood. Many lack the education or the employment skills needed to earn a living, perpetuating generational government dependence. Also impacting is the realization of urban decay, high crime, violence and widespread unemployment.

The youth of this era bear the full burden of every form of human failure: personal, political, social, medical, cultural and religious. This condition is what I have aptly labeled **"AIDS", A**cquired **I**mmune **D**eficiencie**S.** We have contracted **AIDS** in every facet of humanity – weakened, vulnerable and unable to ward off negative influences. It would be pointless to address *the disease* without addressing the **AIDS** of family, church, politics and society that bred it...

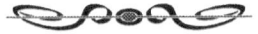

Hillary Clinton wrote a powerful book, *"It Takes a Village"*, detailing the essentiality of involvement and participation in a child's rearing. Today, however, we are at a point that if we could even get a *couple* of villagers that can remember the value of childhood training and rearing, it would make a world of difference – and a different world. The problem lies in the sad fact that many of our seniors, the 'elders' of our village, are left abandoned and languishing though they have a bosom filled with a rich treasure of wisdom and history, readily available to *anyone* who would take time to listen. They were our teachers, our advisors, our confidants who provided instruction to generations, guidance and direction in acquiring essential life-skills. Left alone and longing for even the *slightest* bit of consideration, usually *memories* are all that remains to them of a kinder, gentler day, in which their life was gladly given in sacrifice to 'training up a child in the way he should go.' The abandonment of our seniors is but another characteristic of this self-centered, arrogant, *intolerant* society -- and our *children* suffer the most because of it.

"What's In A Name?"

A name means a great deal more than a lot of people apparently think. Oddly, many names are chosen haphazardly without much thought, at the spur-of-the-moment, or on a whim. However, what you *think* is a really good name might not coincide at all with the personality of your child. A name is a *label* and should say a great deal about the wearer of the label.

I started to write this section under the category of "Verbal Abuse", because I've heard children called by names that couldn't *possibly* mean anything good. I've even heard children called by names that sounded like *cuss* words! A chosen name is the only thing we wear throughout our lifetime. And without knowing the *meaning* of a name, we can place our children at a severe disadvantage early on. Children are teased quite enough without having to bear the burden of a strange name. Since behavior and attitude are tied directly to a person's sense of self-esteem and self importance, the choice of name should not be left to fate or chance. It should be well thought out, discussed and then decided upon. Without knowing a name's meaning we can unwittingly place difficulty in our child's life.

In biblical times, names were chosen at birth that – as it turned out -- *defined* the individual and 'prophesied' their destiny. For example, Naomi named her two sons 'Mah'lon' and 'Chilion', names that actually mean 'weak', 'puny' and 'sickly'. Both sons died very young, leaving two young widows. Names are essential and can dictate your child's future.

Case in point:

My name means 'the bee', which is not much of a depiction. However, what we know about a bee is that it is industrious, busy, diligent, hard-working, focused and meticulous. A bee minds its own business – until you *mess* with it. And guess what? You will *certainly* pay for it! Ask anybody who knows me *at all* and they will tell you that the above characteristics describe me – up to and including the part where if you mess with me or mine, baby, *look out…*

Also importantly, don't assign your child a name that has derogatory significance. Names are important because they may affect a person's behavior. For instance, a name like 'Storm' may be different and it may seem to be a reasonable name choice, *however*, the *implication* is not something you want to be a part of your child's life – or *your* life! Simply because you like the *sound* of it, is not adequate reason to give the name to your child. Rather, choose a name that *you know* has good meaning and one which can be instrumental in bringing blessing upon *everyone's* lifetime.

Names carry a great deal of import. Let us take care to set our children on a *good* path by the name we bestow upon the most precious gift God gives – a baby…

Domestic Violence & Abuse

The very first violent act in human history was an incident of domestic violence involving two brothers, Cain and Abel (Genesis 4:8). Ever since then, mankind has been plagued with all types of domestic violence. There are husbands who batter wives, wives who attack husbands, parents who cruelly beat their children, and grown children who abuse their elderly parents.

The damage caused by domestic violence goes far beyond the physical scars. One battered wife said: "There is a lot of guilt and shame you have to deal with. Most mornings, you just want to stay in bed, hoping it was just a bad dream." Children who observe or experience domestic violence may themselves be violent when they grow up and have families of their own.

Pregnancy, unemployment, the death of a parent, moving, illness, financial problems and taking care of elderly parents bring on stress, as do other things. Most people handle stress without resorting to violence. To some, however, stress can be a prelude to violence, especially when combined with other factors. For example, caring for an aged parent— particularly when the parent is ill—has often led to abuse when the caretaker is overburdened with other family responsibilities.

Raising children produces stress. As a result, the likelihood of child abuse may increase with the size of the family. Children may bring an increase in spouse abuse as well, for "it is conflict over children which is most likely to lead a couple to blows," reports *Behind Closed Doors*.

The most prevalent form of domestic abuse is when men physically assault their wives – hitting, kicking, slapping, or even throwing her against the wall. Some wife beaters suffer from low self-esteem, the same trait they induce in their victims. If they can do that, then their ego will have been fed, and they will feel a measure of superiority and control over another human. They feel that they prove their masculinity in this way. There is a large increase in the number of women being abused over age 50. Many of these older women, even after being physically abused, opt to stay with their abusive husbands, since they will have no other means of financial support and fear being on their own at such an age.

Another example of the unreasonable thinking of the abuser is the fact that he often blames his wife for provoking the beatings. He may imply, or even say to her, such things as: 'You didn't do this right. That's why I'm beating you.' Or: 'Dinner was late, so you're just getting what you deserve.' In the abuser's mind, it is *her* fault.

Many men abuse after drinking. Since alcohol decreases control and raises the potential for acting on impulse, it is not surprising that some feel it can be a catalyst for abuse. Often a person is able to maintain control of violent emotions when he is sober, but after a few drinks, he becomes abusive. The alcohol has dulled his wits and diminished his ability to control his temper.

Others, however, claim that the problem is rooted more in stress than in alcohol itself. They say that a person who uses alcohol to cope with stress is the same type of person who may use violence for that purpose. This means that the drinker may be just as abusive when sober as when intoxicated. Nevertheless, whatever the reasoning in this regard, alcohol is surely not conducive to controlling one's emotions but will usually do the opposite.

Divorce

Nothing has destroyed the moral fabric of society as much as divorce. Many researchers believe that *insecurity in family life* is a major contributing factor in the escalating crime, violence and suicide rate. Divorce has also played a significant role in the dramatic increase in physical, mental and emotional health issues – especially amongst youth. As more and more families are torn apart by divorce, young people are forced to negotiate their own path in an increasingly vicious world, ill-prepared for such a huge undertaking.

Big changes are rarely easy for *anyone*, let alone children and adolescents, particularly when those transitions involve events they can only partially understand. A child of *any* age will have difficulty comprehending why his parents fight, or why one of them no longer lives in the house. Children are forced to choose sides and divide loyalties, even though they love both parents equally. Somehow in all the confusion of separation and/or divorce, the needs of the young child get lost in the shuffle and it is the child who suffers most, experiencing feelings of rejection and abandonment. As a result, some blame themselves for their parents' breakup and decide that their parents would be better off without them. Parental rejection because of family breakup and divorce is a major contributing factor in adolescent suicide.

Aside from the emotional stress that is a part of any divorce, studies show that divorce also accounts for many physical ailments in children and teens. Grief is the prevailing emotion experienced in children when parents divorce. There is a sense of great loss, denial, abandonment and confusion, similar to the death of a loved one. Some children never fully recover, trying continually to win the 'affection' of the absentee parent – and each time re-experience the same pain and rejection when they discover their parents will never be together again. However, rejection has *many* faces…

Child Maltreatment or Abuse

Violence in the home is not limited to spousal abuse, however. Often the assault is directed at the children. Home violence and the maltreatment of a child includes name-calling and shouting, constant criticism, degrading insults, and threats of physical harm and, finally, physical violence.

There are four types of child maltreatment: neglect, physical abuse, sexual abuse, and emotional abuse. Most definitions include the following terminology:

- **Neglect** is failure to provide for a child's basic needs (physical, educational, medical, and emotional).

- **Physical abuse** is physical injury due to punching, beating, kicking, biting, burning, shaking, or otherwise harming a child. Even if the parent or caretaker did not intend to harm the child, such acts are considered abuse when done purposefully.

- **Sexual abuse** includes fondling a child's genitals, incest, penetration, rape, sodomy, indecent exposure, and commercial exploitation through prostitution or the production of pornographic materials.

- **Emotional abuse** is any pattern of behavior that harms a child's emotional development or sense of self-worth. It includes frequent belittling, rejection, threats, and withholding of love and support.

Consequences

- Children who experience maltreatment are at increased risk for adverse health effects and behaviors as adults—including smoking, alcoholism, drug abuse, eating disorders, severe obesity, depression, suicide, sexual promiscuity, and certain chronic diseases (Felitti et al. 1998; Runyan et al. 2002).
- Maltreatment during infancy or early childhood can cause important regions of the brain to form improperly, leading to physical, mental, and emotional problems such as sleep disturbances, panic disorder, and attention-deficit/hyperactivity disorder (DHHS 2001).
- About 25% to 30% of infant victims with SBS (Shaken Baby Syndrome) die from their injuries. Nonfatal consequences of SBS include varying degrees of visual impairment (e.g., blindness), motor impairment (e.g. cerebral palsy) and cognitive impairments (National Center on Shaken Baby Syndrome 2005).
- Victims of child maltreatment who were physically assaulted by caregivers are twice as likely to be physically assaulted as adults (Tjaden et al. 2000).
- Direct costs (judicial, law enforcement and health system responses to child maltreatment) are estimated at $24 billion each year. The indirect costs (long-term economic consequences of child maltreatment) exceed an estimated $69 billion annually (Fromm 2001).

Risk and Protective Factors

A combination of individual, relational, community and societal factors contribute to the risk of child maltreatment. Although children are not responsible for the harm inflicted upon them, certain individual characteristics have been found to increase their risk of being maltreated. Risk factors are *contributing* factors—*not* direct causes.

Examples of risk factors:

- Disabilities or mental retardation in children that may increase caregiver burden
- Social isolation of families
- Parents' lack of understanding of children's needs and child development
- Parents' history of domestic abuse
- Poverty and other socioeconomic disadvantage, such as unemployment
- Family disorganization, dissolution, and violence, including intimate partner violence
- Lack of family cohesion
- Substance abuse in family
- Young, single non-biological parents
- Poor parent-child relationships and negative interactions
- Parental thoughts and emotions supporting maltreatment behaviors
- Parental stress and distress, including depression or other mental health conditions
- Community violence

Protective factors are the opposite of risk factors and may lessen the risk of child maltreatment. Protective factors exist at individual, relational, community, and societal levels.

Examples of protective factors:

- Supportive family environment
- Nurturing parenting skills
- Stable family relationships
- Household rules and monitoring of the child
- Parental employment
- Adequate housing
- Access to health care and social services
- Caring adults outside family who can serve as role models or mentors
- Communities that support parents and take responsibility for preventing abuse

References

Child Abuse Prevention and Treatment Act, Pub. L. 93–247, title I, Sec. 111, formerly Sec. 14, as added Pub. L. 100–294, title I, Sec. 101, 102 Stat. 116 (Apr. 25, 1988); renumbered title I, Sec. 113, and amended Pub. L. 101–126, Sec. 3 (a)(1), (2), (b)(7), 103 Stat. 764, 765 (Oct. 24, 1989); renumbered Sec. 111 and amended Pub. L. No. 104–235, title I, Sec. 110, 113(a)(1)(B), 110 Stat. 3078, 3079 (Oct. 3, 1996). [cited 2002 Jul 1].

Verbal Abuse

Sad, too, is the emotional battering of a child—the constant criticizing and belittling of a child's abilities, intelligence, or value as a person. Such verbal abuse can destroy the spirit of a child – forever. Thousands of teenage youths, now and in the past, have been the victims of what some experts have called a systematic destruction of a youth's self-esteem. Though no bones are broken and no bruises show, ongoing verbal attacks by parents are considered by some to be a very destructive form of child abuse, because it has the potential to cause irrevocable damage to a child's esteem. The wounds of emotional violence are invisible and often go unnoticed by others.

Low self-esteem is not uncommon among youths who are repeatedly called 'stupid' or 'worthless', threatened with violence, made to feel like a failure ("You *never* do anything right!") or constantly blamed for mistakes ("It's all *your* fault!"). Slow mental or emotional growth and destructive or withdrawn behavior are further ill effects attributed by some to verbal abuse. Peer pressure has an extremely prevailing affect on children with low self-esteem. They have the inability to make choices of their own, therefore, tend to follow the perceived leader in order to feel like part of the crowd, to gain a friend and experience a sense of belonging.

Unfortunately, parents make mistakes, too. In the heat of anger, even the *best* of parents occasionally say things they regret. But when harsh, cruel words become a way of life, a destructive pattern results and amounts to serious emotional abuse to the child.

Blair and Rita Justice's study of abusive parents revealed that **85 percent** of them had experienced deprivation and verbal use—if not actual physical abuse—when *they* were children themselves. Therefore, many experts conclude that much of parental abuse comes from the parent's own feelings of insecurity in constructively addressing a situation. Hence, all the old feelings of failure spring forth. Having never received adequate love and nurturing from their own mothers and fathers, some parents find it difficult to deal in a loving manner with their children.

Also, the pressures of making a decent living and of rearing a child in today's society can be overwhelming, to say the least, *especially* for a single parent. It is a fierce cycle of having sufficient employment, securing decent shelter, finding someone trustworthy to keep the children until you get off work, food, etc., etc. And if there's a need to work more than one job to make ends meet, the stress is magnified. Burdened by such pressures, some parents overreact to sometimes even minor infractions committed by the child or teen.

It is highly important that if parents are suffering from emotional difficulties, whether the child is responsible for the problem or not, seek outside help – preferably from a trusted clergyman. It may also be a good idea if the whole family could attend a counseling session of some kind. To be able to discuss and air out grievances together is extremely effective in locating areas that need the most attention. Here's something else that is most effective in crisis prevention or crisis management, and can be done *with* or *without* counseling: PRAY…

Sexual Abuse

Personally, I have never seen quite as many 'nervous' children as I do now and they have ample reason to be. There is so much that goes on in a child's life today. All too often sweet, innocent children have become no more than *by-products* of people's illicit sexual trysts. The two most vital terms used to embody the Godlike responsibilities of parenthood have been unceremoniously diminished to such inconsequential designations as 'my baby Daddy' or 'my baby Mama', with the children caught up in a fierce, absurd rotation of grown people's selfishness, lust and bad decisions.

Sometimes these madcap rendezvous result in a different 'baby mama' or 'baby daddy' for each child. The tragedy of it is we *all* know someone who fits this category – either a man who has babies by two or more different women, or a woman who has children by multiple men… Children are dragged from one place to another, being severed from those to whom they form attachments (although illicit), witnessing abuse, becoming victims of abuse, learning to hate, learning to abuse – it's a tragic truth that happens far too often.

For one thing, many homes are devoid of birth fathers and/or model father figures. There are hardly any reputable and available sources now for children who don't have a father in the home. And many women are making an *even larger* mistake by bringing home 'a man' who is to be the children's 'uncle' or 'play-daddy'. This places children in a precarious situation, for how often is it that we hear heart-rending stories of sexual abuse being perpetrated on young children by 'the man Mama brought home to be my new daddy' – who is in essence, *a stranger*?

Here in St. Louis, I will never forget approximately two years ago when I heard of a young, 28-year old mother of three children, who were all murdered by the man she brought into their home. She was divorced and like many young women, felt the need to have 'a man' around. This young lady had a good job, had a lovely home and three *beautiful* children, ranging in ages from 6 to 11. After many days of not hearing from her daughter, the mother of the 28-year old contacted authorities. She stated that even though her daughter never talked much about what went on in her home, sometimes she would ask her daughter about a black eye, or a bruise she noticed. Her daughter would get defensive and tell her mother to stop butting in her life.

It was discovered by authorities that the children had not been to school in days, and the young lady had not been to work. They found the bodies of all four, in the house, with the air-conditioner on so as to keep the odor down of the badly decomposed bodies.   They had all been shot -- and it was said that the beautiful 11-year old daughter had been kept alive days after her family had been killed -- and molested. It was also discovered that *all* the children had been molested even prior to the killings – even the little 8-year old son.   While the young mother was at work, the *animal* she brought into their home was molesting her children, and would eventually kill them all…

Incest

"She could smell his sweat and foul breath of booze. She felt the roughness of his unshaven face against hers. His body felt so heavy and Rita opened her eyes as he buried his face in her bosom, groaning. She stared through the open window into the night sky, praying to be anywhere but here. Another night, another place, same house. "Maybe Daddy is right, that this is all I'm good at," she thought. Then shutting her eyes tightly, as tears began to run down her face, she silently asked God, "Is this all I'm worth? Is this really what You made me for?" Deep down inside, she hoped not…

During a telephone conversation recently, a friend who works with abused and violent youth stated that the superintendent of the hospital where he is on staff made this shocking remark: "We're going to have to teach the parents *not* to have sex with their children." Even though the remark in itself was disturbing, my friend stated that the *manner* in which the hospital official stated it – plus the fact that he even felt the need to *make* such a suggestion – was beyond belief. Why would parents need to be *taught* not to have sex with children – *their* children? Is the world *that sick*? Unfortunately, yes…

Rita's story is the sad, sad reality of far too many young people -- male and female -- who, as children and through no fault of their own, were taken advantage of by adults and, tragically, many times it is by members of the family. Relationships in later years reflect the abuse of their childhood, being revealed in multiple partners, risqué, licentious sexual activity and prostitution – *always* accompanied with feelings of worthlessness, depression and self-loathing. Intimacy and satisfaction are almost never experienced in subsequent relationships.

The majority of male and female participants in a recent, local survey had been sexually abused as children and preferred a homosexual lifestyle. This is not, however, an implication that *all* homosexuals have been abused, or that everyone abused becomes homosexual, only that there appears to be a strong correlation between sexual abuse (rape, child molestation, etc.), emotional abuse and homosexuality.

But how do you teach a child what love is when their first experience with 'love' was painful, was sordid and set on a confusing, perplexing and *wrong* course? In future relationships, how can one determine or judge what true love is when they have nothing to compare it to? In the world of abuse, especially in the bewildering phase of adolescence, love is given to the first person who validates you by deeming you a desirable *human being* (not a *freak*, not an *animal*), and worthy of love. And in the world of abuse, gender doesn't matter...

Child Permissiveness

Adding to the anxiety and insecurity of young people is 'permissiveness.' Most parents today love their children, and are willing to do whatever it takes to prove it – up to and including giving *children* 'space and privacy'. For all the good intentions of these parents by not 'infringing' upon the rights of their *child*, however, these young people are left feeling alone and in charge of making their own decisions about sex, drugs, alcohol and life in general —decisions they are ill-prepared to make. They see this permissiveness as a lack of love, parental concern and *rejection*. It's a cruel irony that happens far too often in today's society.

Parents, who perhaps have been raised in a strict, disciplined and structured environment, often avow to give their children 'a better life' by allowing them to experience more 'freedom'. Many attempt to befriend their children. A recent study shows that the 'friend' approach is usually taken by mothers who feel this is an effective tool in aiding their teenaged daughters to share their thoughts and emotions.

However, many parents remain heedless and oblivious to what the child *really needs* – love, direction and a *PARENT*. Many children see through the attempt to 'draw them out' and instead of a favorable result, parents can create rebellion, contempt and disrespect in the child. Studies show that children *want* to be parented, have leadership and guardianship – which incorporates love, protection, direction, instruction and discipline.

While parents maintain the need to make a 'better life' for themselves and their children, consider the case of parents who have become so 'busy' outside the home that the children are left to fend for themselves. Rather than considering their parents are attempting to make a better life, all too often children perceive the absence of their parents as neglect and a lack of interest in *them,* which adds to the feeling of rejection.

Also, take for example parents who are rarely at home and who may be totally tied up in their jobs or given to some form of recreation that excludes the children. The indirect message to their offspring is a not-too-subtle rejection. Prominent journalist and researcher Hugh Mackay notes that "parents are becoming more and more self-involved (*selfish*). They put themselves first in order to preserve their lifestyles. . . . To put it brutally, children have gone out of fashion. . . . Life is tough and it all gets a bit self-absorbed."

Young people have an overwhelming need for love and a sense of belonging. Satisfying this need becomes harder and harder in a cold, unfriendly world— which more times than not, sends them 'looking for love in all the wrong places.' Early sex is one of the ways youth attempt to fill the void in their hearts, erroneously associating sex *always* with love. It is devastating when at such a young age these children are in essence 'driven' from their homes in search of love and acceptance, only to experience probable exploitation, abuse, betrayal and rejection from virtual *strangers*, whom these kids confess love for.

Raising Cain – But God Is Able…

During a local 2005 "Eve of Woman" symposium sponsored by one of my sisters, Mrs. Martha West, this topic was used to address 'how to raise a difficult child.' This subject is perhaps the most unsettling issue of parents, especially mothers – how to handle a rebellious child. The first human murder ever committed was done by Cain, the first son of Adam and Eve, who slew his younger brother, Abel, because of jealousy. Evangelist Ruth Nichols, another sister, effectively answered the dilemma: *"Whatever you do, just don't give up on that hard-headed, disobedient, stubborn, black sheep of the family. Love 'em back to life. No matter who says that you should give up – and sometimes you may want to give up – hold on to that troubled child in prayer."*

The evangelist related that *she* was a difficult child, always in trouble. An intravenous drug user for many years, with a multi-hundred dollar a day habit, she related how track marks were even in her *toenails*. She also had an alcohol addiction. *"But Mama never stopped praying for me, even when church folks told her I would never come out of the streets, I was a danger and to have me put away. I remember one night on Sarah and Finney, I had got high earlier and went back to the vacant house. I had sent up this little tin cup on a string with all the money I had for more drugs. This vacant house was a drug house and that's how we did it. You send the money up and they send you back a 'rock' – and sometimes they wouldn't. Well, while standing waitin' for my drugs and being on the lookout, a man walked up on me. In my world, this man was either a cop or somebody trying to steal my drugs. All of a sudden, I heard my mother call, "Ruth Ann?!!!" I turned around so fast and my mind was goin' 'why is Mama down here on Sarah and Finney?' But at the instant I turned and stepped from where I was, there was something that whizzed past my face and I suddenly felt something wet on the side of my head. I turned to ask the man if he saw where Mama went. His face had been blown off! I left that alley not realizing until later that God had used my mother's voice to save my life. He knew she was the only person in the world I would stop for and respond to, because I didn't want her to see me in the shape I was in. God through my mother's prayers saved my life and I'm here tonight to say that even though you are raising Cain, God is able! He's able I tell ya, to give you what to do, how to treat and what to say to that child. But do your part and train that child in the way he or she should go. I'm a living witness that in God's time, He will bring them in!"*

'College' Isn't For *Everyone...*

Hopefully, you'll get the gist of what this title means by the time I'm done with this paragraph. As in preceding paragraphs, most parents want what is best for their children and the last thing we want to do is harm them in any way. However, now and in the past, college has been forced upon many young people, touted as being the *only* way by which an individual can attain a good job, financial security, da-da-da -- whether the youth has been previously able to 'make the grade' or not. There are many, *many* young and gifted youth who barely made it through grade school into high school – and now you want to push *college* off on 'em?

There are three grade categories students fall in: high, middle and low and every parent should know what category their child falls into. What is the point of sending a child to college who has struggled desperately to get even *average* grades in high school but whose mental capacity to *grasp* or *comprehend* hampers his ability to do that?   And it's not that the child is slow or dim-witted, but perhaps only lacks the study skills, test skills, aptitude or necessary propensity for school.

Every child is not college material. The pressure and stress that is added to these youngsters' life is horrific. For not only is the youth aware of his shortcomings in the grade aspect but if the child is of mild temperament, a college environment can be devastating. It's like sending a *lamb* into a *lion's* den. Yet, many parents push their children into going to college because it is the expected thing to do after high school – even though it can have extremely devastating, lifelong consequences. Based on a recent survey, an alarming 1,100 college students take their life each year. Recent studies show an increase in suicides and attempted suicides for college students in general. However, among college freshmen suicide is most prevalent.

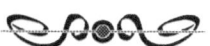

Self-Injury: A Cry For Help...

High-Risk Behaviors – Cutting, Burning, etc.

It is a phenomenon that many parents, grandparents, and guardians of children do not even know exists because it happens behind closed doors and the scars often go unseen: **self-injury**. Can you imagine slicing into your stomach with a razor or carving a design in your arm? Can you imagine burning your fingertips with a cigarette butt or scorching your palms with a lighter? Do you think you could ever *intentionally* break a finger, an arm, a foot, or a leg – just because you *wanted* to?

Self-injury is the act of inflicting physical pain upon oneself for the purpose of relieving or lessening emotional pain or stress, and it is a serious problem among teenagers today. 'Cutting' and other forms of self-injury is an epidemic that seems to be affecting our teens in record highs and in sweeping fashion in America and many countries.

Its basis is psychological and one expert estimates that a mind-boggling **40%** of young people have experimented with some form of self-injury. And once started, many of them can't stop the self-injurious behavior (SIB), self-mutilation, self-abuse, and para-suicidal behavior.

Types of Self-Injurious Behaviors
- Cutting, carving, or slicing skin
- Burning or branding
- Biting or chewing
- Scratching or rubbing to point of abrasion
- Beating, hitting, punching, slapping, or whipping self or objects
- Head banging, hair pulling
- Intentionally breaking bones, or bruising
- Engaging in unhealthy sexual activity
- Excessive body-piercing , or tattooing
- Inserting objects into body cavities

The greatest misunderstanding about SI is the assumption that self-injurers want to die and that their self-injurious behaviors are just masked attempts at suicide. Say the founders of S.A.F.E Alternatives, "Self Abuse Finally Ends", a nationally recognized treatment program, this is not the case. Self-injurers commonly report that they feel empty inside, over or under stimulated, unable to express their feelings, lonely, not understood by others and fearful of relationships. However, in some cases where the injuries escalated and the severity of an injury was misjudged, some teens *have* accidentally committed suicide.

Self-injury is a coping mechanism some people use to get through times of stress, anxiety, conflict, disappointment, or heartache. Self-injury provides relief from the pressure of pent-up feelings. While many do, some self-injurers do not feel any pain when they cut or burn themselves and the prevailing feeling is relief. As one teen put it, "I felt my emotional pain drain away with my blood. It's as though punching a hole in my skin deflated this balloon of intense, overwhelming feelings. Another self-injury explains, "It was like I was dead inside. Cutting reminded me that I was still alive and that I could still feel something."

Some self-injurers are punishing themselves or expressing self-hatred. This is true of those self-injurers who were abused sexually, physically, or emotionally as young children. They replay 'mental messages' they heard from their abusers over and over again: *you're so worthless; it's your fault; you deserve to be punished, you're bad, etc.* In the self-injurer's mind, cutting themselves punishes them with pain and allows them to see some of their 'badness' seep out with their blood.

Suggested Guidelines

- Having someone to talk to in the midst of temptation and turmoil will often help reduce the distress young people may experience during these times: parents, minister (along with the parents), school counselor, etc.
- Teens must seek other means to deal with life's problems, such as, developing hobbies: learn to play a musical instrument, start journaling or painting. Keep mind and body active with *positive* pursuits. Trying self-talk, telling themselves "NO!"
- Making sure they are not alone

Eating Disorders

This is an extremely effective self-harm tool for many young people, who are *desperate* to fit into a cruel, unrealistic ideal the world has created for them. Eating disorders are rampant in our society, causing immense suffering for the victims, as well as their loved ones. Whether by anorexia (starvation), bulimia (bingeing and purging), or extreme overeating, the problem is widespread, complicated and *deadly*. There are also lesser known eating disorders, such as: anorexia athletica (compulsive exercising), pica (craving non-foods like dirt, chalk, paint, etc.), chewing and spitting (not eating or swallowing food), night-eating syndrome (eating most calories at night).

Here are some startling statistics:

•Eating disorders cause immeasurable suffering for individuals and their families.
•Eating disorders have reached epidemic levels in America-- **all segments of society are affected**: *men and women, young and old, rich and poor, all minorities, all socio-economic levels*
•Seven million women
•One million men

Anorexia Nervosa

This intense fear is powerful enough to cause individuals to diet to the point of starvation. While the term anorexia means loss of appetite, this is not true of anorexia nervosa. A person with anorexia is hungry but he or she is afraid to eat because of the fear. Often specific foods are avoided especially those that are high in fat and calories. Often individuals will become vegetarians and want to eat healthily when indeed the issue is the fear of gaining weight.

A person with anorexia constantly thinks about food--how many calories, how many fat grams, how much exercise do you need to do if you eat a cookie, etc. There is always the attempt to try to control eating because of the fear of gaining weight. Often meals are avoided or eaten very slowly, pondering each bite, fearing that surely it will make them fat. These thoughts begin to control a person's mind 24 hours a day, 7 days a week. Your entire life can be centered on this one issue, depriving you of enjoying friends, fun and family.

EATING DISORDER WARNING SIGNS - ANOREXIA NERVOSA

• Deliberate self-starvation with weight loss
• Intense, persistent fear of gaining weight
• Refusal to eat or highly restrictive eating
• Continuous dieting
• Excessive facial/body hair because of inadequate protein in the diet
• Compulsive exercise
• Abnormal weight loss
• Sensitive to cold
• Absent or irregular menstruation
• Hair loss

Bulimia Nervosa

1. Binge Eating

Binge eating in bulimia has certain characteristics that make it much different than an occasional over-indulgence, say at Thanksgiving.

A binge is characterized by:

- A larger amount of food than most people would eat during the same time period (may consist of thousands calories)
- Consumed within a short period of time (typically 2 hours or less)
- A feeling that one CANNOT STOP or CONTROL one's eating
- Accompanied by physical or emotional distress

2. Purging

Following a binge, an individual may feel consumed with fear, guilt or shame and the need to try to undo his/her behavior. Purging is a way to compensate for binging. Purge behaviors come in many forms: vomiting, taking laxatives, water pills, starving or excessive exercise.

Many people in our culture are concerned with how they look, what they weigh or how to change the body parts they don't like. Media messages, fashion images, consumer advertising, toys and television convey a super-skinny image as the norm. In bulimia, there is an intense connection between self-respect and the way the body looks. Even though we seemingly have everything else going our way, if our thighs are too big, well then, we are just not good enough...

EATING DISORDER WARNING SIGNS - BULIMIA NERVOSA

• Preoccupation with food
• Binge eating, usually in secret
• Vomiting after bingeing
• Abuse of laxatives, diuretics, diet pills
• Denial of hunger or drugs to induce vomiting
• Compulsive exercise
• Swollen salivary glands
• Broken blood vessels in the eyes

WHO IS AT RISK OF DEVELOPING AN EATING DISORDER

Females: Because of the increased number of media images portraying 'thin and perfect' models, many girls struggle with body image issues that potentially result in eating disorders.

Youth: Early adolescence to early adulthood with 11 and 17 identified as times for increased vulnerability. Perhaps they represent time of change. The 11 year old may be experiencing changes in her body hormonally as she becomes ready to get her periods. Often there is an increase in fat in 'all the wrong places', creating anxiety. Perhaps it is even *more* difficult when the school -- in a well-meaning attempt to have children be healthy -- measure body fat. Of course, there is always the issue of boys and what culture tells about having an attractive body.

The onset of eating disorders can occur at any age, however, and the age of onset does appear to be getting younger.

Eating disorders can occur at any time and certainly reports of adult onset and individuals at 70 years of age have been reported.

Males: Increasingly, we are becoming more aware of eating disorders in males. For adults, the approximate ratio of men to women is 1:10. About 20-30% of younger anorexics are male. There are probably as many bulimic men than there are anorexic women.

Minorities: Once considered an illness of affluent white females, the picture has dramatically changed. In the US, eating disorders appear to be as common among Hispanic as well as Caucasian women. Recent focus of African American women indicates that it is more common than expected. Black women are prone more to bulimia nervosa and abuse of laxatives. There appears to be an overall increase in other countries.

Athletes: Women participating in certain sports such as gymnastics and distance running are especially vulnerable. Men involved in wrestling are often at risk as they attempt to make weight.

Genetics: Evidence is pointing to the fact that there is a strong genetic component to the illness. There also seems to be some sort of relationship between eating disorders and substance abuse, affective disorders (depression and bipolar) and anxiety disorders.

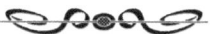

Church AIDS

Church has been central to life, <u>all</u> my life. I can never recall a time when my siblings and I were not a part of the church circuit. Raised by a sweet, quiet father and devout, strict mother we had *absolutely* no choice in the matter and participated in everything from the usher board, to the choir stand, to the pulpit. To miss church was like committing a cardinal sin in my home and I can recall only a couple times in which we did. Church was a house of worship where the presence of God could be felt just by walking through the doors, instilling a sacred sense of awe and reverence.

There were so many great choirs back in the day that we never had a shortage of things to do, or places to go. We would attend three or four church services, musicals, or broadcasts each Sunday and sometimes even more. Christ Southern Mission, Kennerly Temple, Greater Bethlehem, Lively Stone, sometimes Progressive and, finally, back to Kennerly Temple for the Sunday night broadcast. 'The Professor' would make the organ *talk* -- and Bishop Ward never failed to take us to the 'foot of the cross'...

In the past, church was not just a place to go on Sundays but was a 'community center' long before there was a legal definition for the concept. Yes, church was central to life but never more so than within the black community. For it is where we gathered and organized around social and cultural issues, as well as being the place we were taught eternal truths. Many churches served dinner after morning service, had food pantries or soup kitchens and *participated* in the lives of members and non-members alike. In the days of the Civil Rights era and movement, many churches hosted voter registration drives and took an active role in fighting for rights that would better the lives of every individual.

There was a time in bygone days that people could discern that a large family with a recently disabled father and a non-working mother with seven children, had certain needs – and would do everything they could to meet those needs. It was in a time when not only your parents raised you but so did the neighbors, the church mothers, the deacons and anybody else who knew the family you came from. How often did I hear, "You know yo' Mama don't allow that!" They were right... My Mama didn't play. She had it so that when she testified and one of her seven offspring made noise, she would stop in mid-sentence and thump so hard you saw stars, and the sound would reverberate throughout the building.

There was a time when you actually *knew* (and *wanted* to know) your neighbors, when people <u>cared</u> about people and weren't afraid to put love in action. Everybody was involved in your life and upbringing and church was like an extended family, together and sharing whatever we had. I remember outgrowing my eighth-grade graduation dress, which had cost $79 in 1968 – it was soft pink with beautiful floral embroidery around the waist and bell-shaped chiffon sleeves. I wanted to keep that dress forever but Mama encouraged me to give it to a child who *needed* it and who could 'get some use out of it.'

Pastors ministered to the *holistic* need of man. I recall a day when a man could be called a *'great'* man, because the good deeds he did mirrored the type of life he led. It was back in the day when a man could walk into the room and you would catch your breath because of the aura of greatness: Revs. Herman Gore, Sr. and Herman Gore, Jr., Bishop Phillip Lee Scott, Elder F.J. Hayden -- and Deacon Hugh Foster. Deacon Foster was a man of *such* character, faithfulness and refinement -- a deacon of the church for well over *60 years*. When our beloved father passed, my siblings and I 'secretly' adopted Deacon Foster as our dad...

It was a day when men dressed in suits and wore fedoras, and a wino who didn't go to church could recognize a 'man of God' as he passed on the street, stand to one side and remove his tattered hat in respect. Pastors then would stop and take time out to win a lost soul, speak about the love of Jesus and pray, right there on the street. He would then move on to finish his many other *scheduled* appointments – visiting hospitals, homes and prisons.

I can recall a time when a drunk would *stumble* into a church and by the time dismissal rolled around he was able to *walk* out – sober and saved. There were outdoor tent revivals and people would come from miles around, walking across the gravel lot in anticipation of receiving a much-needed spiritual boost. Mama would have us watch the wonderful Dr. Billy Graham on some Wednesday nights (which meant no prayer meeting!)

We always welcomed those times because in the summertime, Mama would tell Andrew to open the door 'so them *devils* up the street can hear', referring to a few of our neighbors -- and *classmates...* On one of these evenings, Betty's high school friend, Shirley, came over to do homework. Dr. Graham was on and, as usual, was speaking of the immeasurable love of God. As we all watched we noticed that Shirley had begun to cry. At the end of the program, at the time when the beloved Cliff Barrows led the choir in *"Oh Lamb of God, I Come"* and at the urging of my mother, Shirley came to God right in my family's middle dining room...

Even though the 1960s was a tumultuous period and when most of the instances I have mentioned occurred, the church had *strength* and was a powerful force, making a positive difference in the world. Madame Fannie Foster and Madame Geneva Gentry conducted 'consecrations' birthed by Rev. Gore. It was not uncommon to run into a group of the saints on a weekday, ministering on the streets or wherever they felt it was necessary, wearing white dresses and prayer caps so white they *glistened.* And if you asked them for prayer, you had better be prepared to *immediately* feel hands on top of yo' head because they would pray for you right where you stood. I had no problem with it but Ruth, Andrew and Mark (if Mama hadn't tied him to a *post* somewhere...) would stand there trying to peek from under their hands to see who was watching and, of course, there *always* would be an amused classmate...

Pastors would preach to parents in their Sunday morning messages to avoid letting their youngsters watch Elvis or the Beatles on the Ed Sullivan show, or to see "The Exorcist" at the movies. I know our pastor Reverend Herman Gore would do it often, thereby possibly averting a great many family crises. Pastor Gore conceptualized a *'Youth Church'* long before it was popular, including youth in *everything* from altar boys to the choirs. They *guided* the flock and didn't mind 'meddling' when it came to giving spiritual direction, always reminding us of what 'thus saith the Lord!' They encouraged their congregants to pray for spiritual and political leaders, and for brave people who were at that time giving their life for noble causes. There was a time when people bragged about their 'church home' because it was indeed like a second home. A person could be born, live 75 or 80 years and die while attending that same church.

But how *unfortunate* it is that the love, compassion and guidance which once existed is missing from society today, and even from our churches, which have become spiritually deficient, anemic and weak. Let me stop here to explain that when mentioning 'church' or 'the church', in these instances I am merely referring to 'a congregation of like-minded people.' Historically, the church was the first line of defense against broken marriages, broken homes and broken lives – effectively preventing the overspill of dysfunction into schools, and other components of society. However, in perhaps the *worst* moral era in the history of mankind the church has become materialistic and *vulnerable,* absent *and* silent in addressing vital social and moral issues.

Many of today's churches have turned into little more than humongous '*members-only*' social clubs and 'costume' parties, filled with narrow-minded, *masked* people craving entertainment. Today, we have multimillion dollar, mega-churches that are so large there's not a *snowflake's* chance that the celebrity pastor will even notice from week to week exactly who is in the congregation – or who is *not*. Many of the members of these churches are so cold and impersonal that friendliness and fellowship -- much-needed essentials in today's society *to cope* -- is not present. Brennan Manning rightly stated, "The institutional church has become a wounder of the healers rather than a healer of the wounded." The church was once a 'hospital' for the sin sick. However, today the sin sick are left on the outside while those who claim to be 'whole' traipse past the wounded, taking up all the hospital beds…

At dismissal nowadays don't expect to greet the pastor at the door, for he is already being whisked away to a waiting limo, airplane, *whatever* – by an entourage of bodyguards and security staff that rival that of Don Carlione's in number and brute force. And if through some miracle a drunk can get anywhere *near* the sanctuary, not only is he man-handled by the on-site security but the local police are called, the FBI, the CIA…

Some argue that times have changed and the church must keep up with the changes in society. Yeah, change *is* necessary… *BUT* can some of the changes *be for better*? Has anybody stopped to consider the fact that the world has actually gotten *much worse* with all the 'changing' and the utilization of modern-day techniques? For instance, some members of clergy are so *busy* that sermons are no longer 'prayed down' but 'pulled off' the internet. Many no longer use the Bible but have replaced it with the latest revised copy of, *"How to Place an Audience in the Palm of Your Hand,"* or some other foolish motivational speaking tool currently being used. Many charge thousands and thousands of dollars to speak at an engagement. Jesus didn't charge the people a *dime* and yet He spoke Words of Life that people are yet talking about today, healed the sick, raised the dead, fed the hungry... The concept of winning souls, which is why church doors stand open in the first place, seems totally lost.

One of the obvious reasons the church has *acquired immune deficiencies* and become so defenseless is that there are more armor-*bearers* than armor-*wearers*! *"For we fight not against flesh and blood, but against principalities and powers; against spiritual wickedness in high places"* (Ephesians 6:11). Does this sound like the time to let someone else carry your war clothes? The church has become *unfortified*, unprotected. Paul used the analogy of the Roman army, recorded in history as a most formidable opponent, to systematize the army of God with the necessary equipment and apparel to combat the devil.

The first piece of armor the Word talks about is 'having our loins girdled about with truth. In battle this is an obvious, effective target of the enemy. If you don't have on the girdle, there is *no support* and *no protection* for the midriff and *groin* area. *All that's* hangin' out. And anyone knows that if you are hit in *that* sensitive area, honey, the fight is *over* before it even got started... You don't even *want* to fight after being hit in *that* spot! (Naw, just let me lay here and *die,* okay?...) This is where the devil first attacks -- our sex organs -- the area that is *extremely* sensitive, vulnerable and the part of us we more readily surrender without a struggle. Also, without the girdle there is *no place* to put your sword.

Put on the helmet of salvation to protect your mind! *Put on* the breastplate of righteousness to protect your heart (emotions)! *Shod your feet* for swiftness in bearing the gospel! *Take up* the shield of faith to ward off the fiery darts of the enemy, and *pick up* the sword of the Spirit: the Word of God. '*Put on the WHOLE armor of God that you might be able to withstand in this evil day, having done all to stand*!

Some of these often vacillate on the applicability and practicality of some Scriptures, at times favoring the New Testament over the Old

Testament and at other times, vice versa. By instituting this method of vacillation, many of the basic tenets and rudiments of the church -- such as Holy Communion and feet-washing (which implies *service* and *humility*) -- have been dismissed as outdated (New Testament) and replaced with ineffective practices and policies instituted by some pastors.

However, these tenets are *foundational* and were instituted by Jesus Christ, who they claim to be servants of. Jesus said to his disciples or servants, *"If I then, your Lord and Master, have washed your feet, you also ought to wash one another's feet. I have given you an example that you should do as I have done. Truly, truly, I say to you, the servant is not greater than his lord; nor is he that is sent greater than he that sent him"* (John 13: 14-16). How can it be any plainer? Today, however, these 'servants' own nearly commercial-sized aircraft, mansions, *fleets* of cars -- and Jesus Christ, the son of God, had nowhere to lay His head. . .

Is there any wonder about the extreme breakdown of society? Has anyone considered that we have *more want, more lack* and *more need* than ever before? The divorce rate is at an all-time high of over 50%. The crime rate is staggering. There are more homeless *families* than ever before. There are more single mothers and grandparents raising small children than at any other time in history. There are more young people who *yet* mourn the death of Tupac and Biggie Small – but have never heard about Jesus' death on their behalf. There is something *desperately* wrong with this picture of churches having become larger but even *less effective* than the much smaller churches of yesterday, who in their *crudity* managed during the Great Depression to feed the hungry, provide jobs and shelter, keep families together, provide effective direction -- and touch people in every faction of life.

God knows there are enough of them. In St. Louis there are at least two churches on every block, many churches that are across the street from each other and some that are even directly *beside* each other. With the sheer numbers of churches present in our neighborhoods there is no excuse whatsoever for *anyone* to be hungry, homeless, without employment and ignorant concerning what the Bible states on *every* issue that plagues humanity. It appears that with the enlargement of the contemporary church that its heart and mind have become so small.

Minister Samson Latchison, my brother, who does a vital work with troubled and violent youth, made this profound statement: "Is the church ready to realize the delicate juxtaposition of our reality and God's truth? The church is not immune to the devastation of AIDS… it has lost some of its finest musicians, ministers and teachers… Yet the church has worn a blindfold of pretension … her freshly-washed hands dripping with blood … her feet firmly placed on doctrines and protocol."

What is the church's place in the world today, if not to address the issues facing people – not people *globally* – but people who live in the same community and make up the congregation? Brighten the corner where *you* are! If *every church* that professes to adhere to the teachings of Jesus Christ would display the same love and concern that He did in addressing the needs of man, there would be no lack. One prominent bishop has stated, "Compassion is a *divine* trait… its source lives in a more foundational emotion – love that is *agape*. Compassion is crucial for genuine ministry, although this emotion is not readily present… not even in the church".

Jesus, the Son of God, walked among the people and met their every need. Multitudes followed Him when He taught (e.g., the Sermon on the Mount) and though the disciples wanted to send the people away hungry, Jesus had compassion and fed them. When the leper said to Jesus, "If you want to you can make me clean." Jesus said, "I want to" and touched the leper, who immediately became whole. Jesus gave everyone what was needed for *each situation.* In other words, he didn't feed the leper and touch the multitude. The multitude *needed* to be fed, the leper *needed* to be touched.

The church must come up with practical solutions to suit the problem. Some may say that we have no leprosy in this modern society, or in this country but even though many claim to go to the nth degree for people in Africa with AIDS, virtually none have embraced the cause of the epidemic's toll in America. And these people experience the same isolation and 'untouchability' from church people that lepers did from the Pharisees in biblical times.

There's a huge increase in the number of churches constructing more expansive edifices to accommodate the large crowds of *already* church-going people. However, even though many of these newly constructed churches are the size of a *football* field, they don't allow plans for even enough space to house a *food pantry* to give a bag of groceries to people in the surrounding community. I saw a recent commercial that poignantly stated that a person does not have to leave their own country to find third-world poverty. I whole-heartedly agree but will go a step further to say **we do not have to leave our own *city* to find third-world poverty.** The 'mission field' is everywhere you look...

Has anyone thought about just going out onto the *street* and taking the message of God's love and salvation? Prisons, senior care facilities, orphanages, hospitals – all these institutions are *filled* with people that are *desperate* to receive the Good News. Jesus said, *"Inasmuch as you have done it unto one of these my brethren, you have done it unto me"* (Matthew 25:40).

Far be it from me to say that *every* church is guilty of avoiding community-mission. Recently, I heard of a wonderful church in Florida who is actually 'a church without walls', doing a vital, holistic work on a huge scale – attracting motorcycle gangs and those who wouldn't step foot in a traditional church. *"And the Lord said, Go* <u>out</u> *into the highways and hedges, and compel them to come in"* (St. Luke 14:23). This type of effective ministry should be the focus of the 21st century church. However, for the most part, even churches whose *name* is 'The Church without Walls' *have walls* and lack the fortitude to come from behind those walls and into the world, where people are *dying*. It is clear that the whole *world* needs much more 'uninstitutionalized' church development, activity and involvement.

James 2:14:17 says (paraphrased), *"What does it matter, my brother, if a man says he has faith but has nothing to back it up with? If a brother or sister be without clothing and destitute of daily food, and one of you says to them, 'Go in peace, be you warmed and filled' but haven't given those things that they are needful of, what good is your faith? Faith without action is dead, being alone."*

Speaking of being *alone*, that is exactly what *anyone* is who even suggests coming 'out of the box.' It seems that church members get *phobic* at the mere *mention* of plans to 'go out into the community' -- which by the way is approached with the *same* concentration, intensity and strategic planning that it takes to build *and* launch a spaceship! Perhaps 20 out of a membership of 5,000 may 'volunteer' but act as if they pulled the short straw for a *kamikaze* mission. We need to just *get out there*, for Pete's sake – and Paula's sake, for Jerrod's sake and Donna's sake. And I don't mean just once a year, or once every other Saturday/Sunday because when the time *finally* comes, e'erbody has something else they need to do. ("Well, sister, you *do* know that we only have *one* Saturday/Sunday every blue-moon-Haley's-comet-eclipse-leap year, don't ya? I mean can't you just *wait* until some other time to do what you..."). You're standing there talkin' to the person's *back* because they have *long* since walked off...

If you *must* build a building, then build a building that builds people: a hospital, a school, an orphanage, a senior assisted-living facility... James 1:27: '*True religion and undefiled before God is this: to visit the orphans and widows in their destitution and to keep yourself untarnished from the world.*'

Today, in a world where 'minister' is nothing more than a title and the word 'outreach' is part of the name of a church, it is high time that we make these words become *action* words. **Minister**: comfort, attend to, look after, care for, nurse, wait on. **Outreach**: reach *out*... to the disenfranchised, to the lost, the hungry, the homeless, the spiritually, physically, mentally and emotionally infirmed. Reach out to those with AIDS... And if you reach out, you're bound to touch *some*one.

Many things are broken today -- broken homes, broken families, broken people, broken lives and shattered dreams. Such are the sad consequences when you build buildings without building people...

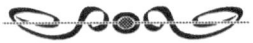

Political AIDS

This will be an exercise to determine your skill in the area of political perception. Below are listed several possible options and you are to choose the answer(s) that best define the word "politics". Carefully think your answers through before making your selection and if asked, be prepared to defend your choices by providing discourse.

Politics: What Does It Mean?

(A)   When heads of nations use the lives of their constituents as pawns in cruel games of war, money and power

(B)   When several methods are utilized to commit genocide

(C)   When it is stated in a given month that the 'economy is improving', even though five major companies have laid off a total of over 100,000 individuals

(D)   When a candidate can win an election based on an 'overwhelming majority of votes' in a certain district or city, even though overflowing ballot boxes lay abandoned and votes *uncounted*, at the very 'district' that allegedly put the candidate over the top

(E)   When after an act of terror, a 'leader' *vowed* to capture one man but instead declared war on another, *dropping bombs* on 'weapons of mass destruction'. (Be prepared to discuss methods which can be utilized to capture a tall, crippled, bearded man whose features are relatively ambiguous, due to the grainy footage on which he always appears. Also discuss the fact that though it is said to be difficult to capture this man, he always appears as if 'cued' just after the leader warns: "This country is expecting a terrorist attack during the election period." And the day before the election, the man appears – again on grainy footage -- as if to 'corroborate' what had been stated ('Yeah, like he said yesterday, I plan to...'). Cite other instances wherein it appears O'Someone Bin Lyin'...

(F)   None of the above

(G)   All of the above

After completion, submit this exercise to Yo' Conscience for grading.

It seems that more now than ever before we are experiencing a massive number of disasters, many of them 'natural'. Hurricanes, tornados, floods and famines -- all of these have brought extreme personal, financial, physical and emotional suffering. Who will ever forget the tsunami, or Hurricane Katrina and the *horror* it brought to Alabama, Mississippi and Louisiana victims? In the aftermath of the city of New Orleans laid *bare* by the raw fury of a hurricane, mothers are yet searching for their children, husbands and wives are yet apart, wondering if the other survived, homes will never be rebuilt and so many others are forever traumatized at the horrors they beheld...

"There were dead babies in the water all bit up by snakes and turtles. And I saw a family that was all joined together like they were hugging, but they were all dead."
Ron'jana, 8, about what she remembers – Essence Magazine, November 2005

One two-word question hauntingly and heavily weighs, not so much on the mind as on the *heart* of the human community: *What happened? What happened* that there was such an enormous absence of official preparation and intervention? *What happened* that there was such a lack of compassionate response by the government to the *worst* human disaster on our soil? *What happened* that this country allowed the barely-living, narrowly-escaped and nearly-dead to languish even longer in sweltering heat, fetid and diseased water, in urine and feces – beside the newly dead? Dependent on government assistance and hence the reason many stayed behind, they were starving *long before* Hurricane Katrina...

"When we got to Jefferson Parish we were hopeless, hapless, hungry and hurricaned out, and what did we have to greet us? Military police with M-16 rifles. They watched us, caged us in barricades, laughed at us, and took pictures of us with their camera phones. This was murder. They wanted us to die..."
Alva, 58, taken from New Orleans to Houston - Essence Magazine, November 2005

With all that happened to that essential portion of our land, cruel insults and insensitive statements were made regarding the devastation and the devastated:

"These people were extremely poor… they didn't have much to begin with. So really the Dome is more than they're used to…"

"You did a helluva job, Brownie!"

"Diane, there is an absolutely zero tolerance policy for looting. All looters will be punished to the fullest extent"…

They said, 'We can't rescue you unless you get to your roof.' I said, 'I can't. I have two children and an elderly motherly in a wheelchair'. They said, 'If you don't get up there, we'll just throw down some body bags and you can zip yourselves in'…

~~~~~~~~~~~~~~~~~~

"Be not deceived, God is not mocked. *Whatsoever* a man soweth, *that* shall he also reap…" (Galatians 6:7)

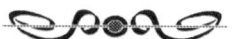

Societal AIDS

"And because wickedness shall be in abundance, the love of many shall grow cold" (Matthew 24:12)

In this country even during tumultuous periods, I am sure we can all evoke wonderful memories of happier, though much simpler, times. Do you recall Sunday drives after church, bike riding, eating watermelon on the porch, catching fireflies, merry-go-rounds, flying kites, building wagons, family gatherings, drinking water from a hose, sunny-day picnics, climbing into the small inflated pool on hot days, looking up into a starry sky, picking wildflowers, bird-watching, collecting soda bottles to cash in for five cents apiece, hearing the early-morning hawking of the paperboy, or the fish, fruit and vegetable men, selling wares from their trucks?

In comparison to what we have today, the times were crude. We didn't have Playstations, Nintendo's, X-boxes, video games, no 150 channels on cable, no video movies or DVDs, no surround-sound or CDs, no cell phones, no personal computers, no Internet or chat rooms. WE HAD FRIENDS TO PLAY WITH – AND WE WERE HAPPY! Those were the good ole' days when you could get together, go to the corner store and buy a Big Time or Payday candy bar for five cents, a Hostess cupcake for 12 cents and 'penny' candy for actually *a penny*! It is hard to believe but it was not that long ago when you could pick up the phone, call someone and actually get a *real, live person* on the other end to interact with – not a machine…

Today, however, as Joan Puls once wrote: "We refrigerate ourselves in summer and entomb ourselves in plastic in winter. We rake up every leaf as fast as it falls. We buy pre-packaged meats and fish and fowl in supermarkets, without thinking or blinking about the bounty of God's creation. We lead practical lives. We miss the experience of awe, reverence, and wonder." (*"A Spirituality of Compassion"*, Mystic, Conn.: Twenty-Third Publications, 1988). As a result, we miss *life*…

In recent years there has been an obvious death of the heart of the people of this country. Everyone's bottom line seems to be 'the all-mighty dollar' — getting it at any cost, by any means necessary... There is tension, restlessness – and *crime*. What happened to the Golden Rule of 'do unto others as you would have them do unto you?' The fact is we have become exceedingly preoccupied with *ourselves*, our jobs, our plans that we perceive to be much more important than human relationships. It is largely to blame for our selfishness and impatience. We have become so *unfeeling*, so intolerant and completely indifferent as to whether others are making it.

We don't have time any longer to take notice of things that at one time tugged at our heart strings, which prompted us to give something or say a whispered prayer: a street beggar, a young mother with children who has been evicted, someone who has lost a good job, an elderly person who ran out of money for food and has to put back a few essentials. Nowadays, there are those who make a *career* of preying on the street beggar, the disenfranchised and the elderly – robbing them of what little they have. We have become arrogant, remote and *desensitized*.

But if only we could walk in some other's shoes, perhaps we could *then* become more compassionate. Recently, we lost the Pope and his *beautiful* legacy of love and unprecedented display of compassion in the world. All over the world, his message was to get people to see that we are not *so* different. If only we could just for a moment forget who we are and what we have and just imagine what life is like for someone else who doesn't have what we have. No one should have less than I have for if I give you half of mine, we have equal.

We really don't help *anyone* if our motive is not just to help *some*one. What is the difference between one homeless man from another, or one hungry man from another? If our only objective is to feed the hungry, what is the difference between feeding the hungry in Africa, from feeding the hungry in *America*? What is the difference between adopting an orphaned child in another country, from adopting an orphaned child in America – if the intent is just to provide a child a loving home? Why do we reach clear across the world to help those there and yet completely disregard the destitution, squalor and third-world conditions present even in *our own city*? Yes, help those in Africa but also in America. Yes, help those in China but also India. There is plenty to go around for *everyone*...

If we would try to feel what others feel when we hate them because of the color of their skin, their social status, or economic bearing, then by and large this world would regain its ability to be fascinated by something other than violence and evil. This world would regain its love and tolerance.

The profound Minister Louis Farrakhan stated aptly in a 1992 sermon in Chicago, Illinois: "By being estranged from God, it is only natural that we would be estranged one from another, each one glorying in their sect. I'm a Christian; I'm a Muslim; I'm Orthodox; I'm Sunni; I'm Shiite; I'm educated, you are not; my hair is straight, yours is nappy… We really get wrapped up in ourselves. The whole theme is 'I am better'. Allah (God) didn't create any of this. We did this to one another. Now, we are all divided by race; we are divided by sex; we are divided by nation; we are divided by language. We have become a great Tower of Babel". ("*The Oneness of God"*, The Final Call, January 2007).

In his book, "The Magnificent Defeat," Frederick Buechner wrote: "What we need to know, of course, is not just that God exists, not just that beyond the brightness of stars there is a cosmic intelligence that keeps the whole show going, but that there is a God *right here* in the thick of our day-to-day lives who may not be writing messages about Himself in the stars but in one way or another is trying to get messages through our blindness as we move around down here knee-deep in the fragrant muck and misery -- and *marvel* of the world". We need to know this so desperately…

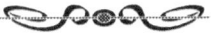

Blacks have endured kidnap, rape, murder, torture, slavery, hunger, disenfranchisement – and we're *still* here. Our men in horror and pain have heard the sound of his dismembered perpetuation, in the past and in the present. With heads lifted towards the heavens we have heard the roar of our own agony, fear and anger deep within, as our families were and are dismantled. But yet we remain – for at one time we realized our very existence was connected to the God of the Universe. It's been said that 'you can't kill us with a *meat cleaver*.' It has been proven that blacks are perhaps the most indomitable race of people that has ever survived. It seems that the *only* thing that will be our undoing and the reason for our total extinction – is *us*…

We have veered so far from the path laid by our forebears, that if we do not *soon* find it again, it will be too late. It is *high time* that we return to our *roots*, to the values, heritage and legacy left to us by the people who took an active part in our life and in creating a safe haven for us -- our parents and grandparents, teachers, pastors, spiritual and respectable leaders. Recently, we lost two very important icons to our struggle -- Rosa Parks and Coretta Scott King. Each in her manner maintained the 'backbone' necessary to persevere in a difficult, dangerous period. We boomers remember that period and understand fully the sacrifices made and the guts it took to make them. But I wonder did we appreciate those life-sacrifices as much as we *should* have?

After Mrs. Rosa Parks' selfless act of courage for her people, did we make her life *the best* it could have been? If we were to admit the truth as painful as it is, unfortunately no – but we *could* have, *should* have made it much better. Immediately after she did what she did, her life and the lives of her husband and mother were constantly threatened and Mrs. Parks had to leave her home. In old age, someone broke into her home in Michigan, robbed and beat her. At one time she was even threatened with eviction, when it was said that the landlord had not received payment from Mrs. Parks' custodian. And even though it was later corrected to the point she never had to pay rent again, I can only imagine the fear and trauma she must have experienced.

When she died *millions* lauded and applauded her, as well we should have. But although she was placed in the nation's Rotunda and leaders from all parts of the globe paid respects, I can't imagine that she knew anything about it. We have made many people in this country *rich* whose contribution to society couldn't come *close* to that of the essential Mrs. Parks – and though she might have been *comfortable,* she honestly deserved so much more…

The beautiful Mrs. Coretta Scott King, who with quiet dignity, stood stoically by her man through *thick* and *thick* – marching, sittin'-in, *fighting* for the rights of a people beside her husband, Dr. Martin Luther King, Jr. Yet the boomers, who watched, fought and *knew* the struggle allowed the *one place* designated to pay tribute and respect to a great man's life and sacrifice, be sold to the Parks Dept. What are we *doing,* if we can't honor and hold together the sacred inheritance passed on to us by our predecessors to guard and cherish? Dare we extinguish the eternal flame of *hope*? We have *failed* to teach our children the power of perseverance in a struggle for rights in which we believe. We have failed to impart *their* history by failing to tell them of *our* history. Yes, we need a return to our life-subsisting and life-sustaining roots, to those things foundational, essential and eternally true, for our very existence...

Speaking of *roots*, our elders possessed a trove of God-given knowledge regarding the medicinal benefits of roots, natural herbal cures that are effective and do not produce the side-effects and other risks associated with traditional medicines. There was a day when you didn't hear about all the ailments that people are today stressed with, especially people of color. It appears that *everyone* has diabetes, high blood pressure, heart trouble, cancer, strokes – or any combination of these illnesses and more. But the ancestors *knew* something back in the day which enabled them to fend off sicknesses, despite the fact their diet consisted heavily of pork. Back then no one had trouble with their cholesterol level.

My dear mother had a special passion for oatmeal, which I consider an indispensable food. Though she reared seven children, not a single one of us *ever* spent a day in a hospital for broken limbs, assaults or sickness – and we were some pretty tough cookies. For colds, it was 'Three Sixes' (666), Father John cold medicine (which Ruth would slip and drink like *water*), or castor oil with baking soda and sugar in it. For vitamin, she would give us cod liver oil and by the time my younger siblings came along, Flintstone's chewable tablets were available. After each of my younger siblings was born, Mama would wrap a piece of a torn sheet tightly around her waist in order to keep her 'waist down'. Tall and elegant, she kept her shape almost until the day she died, at 71 years of age in 2000.

Mama had no problem pulling out the bottle of Pompeii olive oil which she would have our pastor to pray over, and slick us down with it. And it *worked...* She had no problem buying a box of unsalted crackers and a bottle of Welch's grape juice, to give herself Holy Communion. And it *worked...* Doctors had given her up to die since she was 36 years old due to bone cancer, an enlarged heart, high blood pressure, congestive heart failure, angina and any number of other ailments doctors discovered before she died.

God gave our ancestors *wisdom*, or mother-wit, though most never went to college and some were never taught to read. They knew how to mix herbs and spices in various brews and teas, in foods, made medicines, salves and ointments – all with roots. They prayed, fasted, and didn't have all the weight issues we have now. They *walked* nearly everywhere they went – so *there's* the exercise! We need to stick with the tried and true. There's no need to reinvent the wheel. If it worked for them, it will work for us.

With hospitals assailed with all types of disease and infections (staphylococcus), I would *much* rather take advice from someone who has lived 75, 80, 85 or 90 years than from someone whose handwriting I can't read, can barely make out what is being said -- and who by his own admission is just 'practicing' medicine...

There was something else that worked for us in the past: *gospel music*. Songs of the church like 'Precious Lord, Take My Hand,' 'Amazing Grace', 'There is a Fountain', 'Love Lifted Me', etc. are songs that got us *through*. *Right now*, when somebody sings 'There Is a Fountain' and get to the verse: *'The dying thief rejoiced to see that fountain in his day; and there may I, though vile as he, wash all my sins away'* -- honey, somebody will be picking me up off the *flo'*...

In the day when Rev. James Cleveland was 'The King' of gospel music and Shirley Caesar sang, 'God is Not Dead', The Caravans, Mahalia, Clara Ward, Roberta Martin, Goldie and Rosie Haynes, Rev. Charles Nicks, Rev. Clay Evans, St. Louis' O'Neal Twins and Rev. Cleophus Robinson, Sr. – all of these got us through the 60s and beyond. Later, the fantastic Andre' Crouch came out with 'Jesus Is the Answer' – a song so basic and yet so profound that it touched a *world*. There was the unforgettable Hawkins Family: 'Goin' Up Yonder,' 'Follow Me', 'A Change' – *all* fantastic hits. There were great choirs like the Thompson Community Choir, the Milton Bronson Singers and the wonderful, late Thomas Whitfield.

But of all the marvelous singers mentioned, my personal favorite *of all-time* is *The Winans: Marvin, Carvin, Michael and Ronald* (and Lord, don't we miss *Ron?* A whole *lot* of us are missing that sweet Heart…) *Every*one ought to have *some*one on this earth they can look to for inspiration – and since October 1982, The Family has been mine. (When I get the chance I'm going to ask that angel Mom where she keeps her wings – and *wonder*ful Pop: *'He's a Wonda, aint' he?'*) My children were *raised* on their music, could probably name any tune in three notes *and* tell you which album it's on. And anytime it was even *rumored* they were going to be somewhere, we'd be like hippies trying to get to Woodstock… Like boomers tryin' to see the Grateful Dead in a final concert. Car, bus, plane, hitch-hiking – it didn't matter – we'd get there so fast it was like we were *beamed.* We would ask people on the streets of Detroit and this is how the conversation would go: **Me/Charles:** "Uh, will any of the Winans Family be in concert or preachin' anywhere?" **The Detroit Person:** "No, not this week but next week…" **Me/Charles:** "Okay, we be back"… The Family has made such *powerful*, profound music it makes you stop and think: 'Now how did they come up with *that*?' Apparently, they *stay* in the Throne Room. It has always been about God with them. They have never failed to carry the good news of the Gospel wherever they go. And *that* has been what has saved countless lives. I know it saved *mine*…

There are many wonderful new gospel artists that are effective in their endeavors to reach younger audiences, adding 'extra flava' using enhanced instrumentation. However, I would have to agree with a well-known comedian on a recent BET awards program, who remarked about the power and essentiality of traditional gospel music: "If I'm hangin' over a cliff, I need to hear some 'Precious Lord, Take My Hand', or 'Amazin' Grace'. I'm sorry, but some of this music they makin' now ain't gon' help me…" Just because something is 'new' doesn't always mean it is *'improved'*…

Family, we need to stop pretending that we know nothing about God, about church. I know that *every* black individual knows about church -- from rap artists to rock stars to actors to strippers to *crack*heads. Many of today's most well-known artists, singers and musicians got their beginning in church, singing in the choir. *Despise not small beginnings.*

Our mothers and grandmothers took us to church and taught us by example how to live principled lives. They believed in God even when things were at their worst: slavery, segregation, lynchings, raw prejudice, the Great Depression, no jobs, famine and war. Even in the roughest times they *yet* prayed, they still shouted -- they *believed* and made it through. Though they didn't possess *knowledge*, which comes from 'book-learning,' God endowed them with wisdom, which is but *common sense*. *"If any man lack wisdom let him ask of God that gives to all men liberally, and upbraideth not"* (James 1:5).

There's really no need to get all complicated or sophisticated in our thinking about God. It's all really quite simple: *"In all of your ways acknowledge God and He shall direct your path"* (Proverbs 3:6). We need to stop letting this world dispel our belief in the existence of Almighty God. Denying does not make Him *not exist*.

It has been said that a man who knows not his past, knows not himself. It has also been said that those who fail to *learn* from the past are doomed to repeat it. I feel the black race of people in this country is now repeating the most tragic part of our history: enslavement. This time, however, we are not enslaved by any particular race or creed -- but rather by our own selfishness in the fulfillment of dangerous passions, by any means. We have been arrogant in assuming that the adoption of certain behaviors would not bring reprisal.

Many blacks have taken for granted the enormous sacrifices made by great, *peerless* leaders to the extent younger generations know nothing of their valuable legacy. Their selfless acts of determination, hard work, time and faith in God were the elements utilized to bring us to this present place. However, for all that was accomplished by those great men and women, it will not go down in perpetual history that a race of people died nobly, attempting to protect that legacy. Neither will their demise have been caused by unavoidable flood nor famine, as in other extinct civilizations. Instead, it will be said for time eternal that the African-American race of people came up absent from the planet as a result of their arrogance, selfishness, lack of discipline, sexual irresponsibility and indiscretion – from a sexually transmitted disease: **AIDS**...

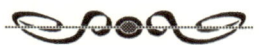

Suicide

In the United States there are some 25,000 suicides recorded each year. There is also estimated to be an accumulated total of several million persons who have tried to take their lives. Some countries have even higher suicide rates than the United States. Worldwide the suicide rate has reached alarming proportions. Both the wealthy and the poor are involved—and the numbers keep increasing. Psychiatrists attribute this increase to a number of things – from poverty, to loneliness, to extreme illness. The most striking increase in suicides and suicide attempts, however, is among youth. In the United States some sources estimate that 57 children and teenagers attempt suicide *every hour*. Canada has had a fourfold increase in young suicides since the 1950's. In Canadian youth ages 10 to 24, suicide is the second leading cause of death, and the third leading cause of death for the same age group in the United States. Similar trends are reported from France, the Federal Republic of Germany, Japan and Sweden.

Unfortunately, teen suicide rates appear to be rising. More kids seem to be taking their lives, or attempting to do so, each year. But why do so many young people feel unable to cope with life? *Hopelessness about the future* is pointed to as one of the leading reasons. Dr. Diane Syer, as director of the Crisis Intervention Unit at Toronto's East General Hospital, said that young people who attempt suicide sense "that their world isn't going to get any better and so what's the use of going on." Depression, hopelessness, helplessness, school pressures (grades, being bullied, etc.), low self-esteem, sex abuse and substance abuse, are all emotions that can make an individual pursue self-destructive coping mechanisms.

Complicating the issue of suicide amongst teens is the inability to think in the 'big-picture'. Whatever they're currently experiencing seems that it will go on forever. Some teens can't imagine that things will work, or get better. A sad example is when parents divorce and the child or teen can't imagine life without *either* of them. Or if a teen makes a failing grade, they know they can't live with the pain or disappointment forever. Sadly, this short-sighted perspective leads the hurting child or teen to take a permanent route to solution: they end their lives... Another factor is the *devaluation of life,"* says Dr. Herbert Hendin, associate clinical professor of psychiatry at New York City's Columbia University. "By the time a child is 15, he or she has witnessed 14,000 murders or violent deaths on television," says Dr. Seiden. Added to this are the popular songs that glamorize suicide in theme: *"Think I'm Gonna Kill Myself"*; *"I'm Mortuary Bound"*; *"Suicide."*

To help someone see beyond suicide you must first recognize whether or not they really are suicidal. We all get depressed and blue now and then. And it's perfectly normal to be sad when you lose someone near and dear to you. Sadness and depression don't necessarily lead to suicide. However, a suicidal person will experience these same emotions but he or she will also exhibit other signs, such as expressing the desire to die, talking about death, having a suicide plan, has suicide ideations (methods of suicide), giving away personal belongings, suddenly seeming happier or calmer (resigned) after having been severely depressed. If you or a loved experiences any of these warning signs, seek help immediately. Call a religious leader, a teacher, a coach or any other trusted adult. Call 911 or take the person to the nearest emergency room if your friend lays out the plan for you. Also, the U.S. National Suicide Hotline is 1-800-SUICIDE and is a toll-free number. Save a life – whether it's your life or someone else's.

Gang Activity

"As I sat in the locker room at school, these guys came up to me and began to bother me. One of them punched me in the chest. At that point one of the guys I knew from the gang in my neighborhood came over and took up for me. I thought to myself, 'If I join the gang, maybe I can have protection like this.'" —Greg.

Gangs are a growing presence and police estimated in 1996 that in Los Angeles County, U.S.A., alone there were 600 gangs, with some 70,000 members. Gangs are not limited to the United States, however. England, Spain, Canada, Germany, South Africa, Brazil – the problem is no longer confined to certain regions. Like Greg, many join gangs to gain protection from school violence and in these violent times, it is not difficult to understand why some youths may feel such a need. We are witnessing a worldwide "increasing of lawlessness." (Matthew 24:12) However, there are yet other reasons why street gangs hold such a powerful attraction for some youths – friendship and support.

"*I really wanted to have friends, a sense of belonging to somebody or to a group, somebody you could care for,*" explains Bernard, a former gang member. Marianne, who joined a girls' gang, admits that she did so "*out of [her] need to control something,*" as well as for the "*family atmosphere*" it offered. While it is true that some youths join gangs to help deal with boredom or for the excitement they might offer, it appears that far more join to have a sense of belonging, to receive emotional support, to get friends with whom they share things in common. Often this is done to replace an undesirable family situation.

Bernard says of himself and fellow gang members: "*Most of us came from broken homes. Many were being raised by a single parent, usually a mother, in large families. So there was no one to take time to talk to us. Many came from homes where they were physically and verbally abused and where no one cared whether we had feelings or not. So it felt good to talk to someone and be heard.*" This point is also made by Canadian youth counselor Lew Golding. He stated: "*Kids having problems at home latch on to a gang for emotional nurturing.*"

In the United States, many gangs are formed along ethnic or cultural lines. Gangs in that respect offer the additional appeal of association with those who share feelings regarding food, music, language, and a host of other things. For youths and adults alike, the desire to feel needed and accepted is normal. However, in the high-pressure environment in which gangs operate, grudges easily develop. Disagreements and violent fights among fellow gang members are all too common. Also, differences of opinion can be interpreted as disloyalty. Bernard relates: "*If we had an argument, I had to be on the alert because all of a sudden, a knife or a gun could come out. And these were supposed to be my friends! Gang life left me disappointed because I had no real friends.*" As one other 18-year-old gang member adds: '*You don't have any friends, not even in your own gang. You are by yourself...*'

Among the problems listed as reasons why youth become associated with gangs was inadequate family life, poverty, deteriorating neighborhoods, and poor education. Gang activity has not helped this situation at all, nor has it really helped lonely youths to find genuine friendships...

The Foster Care System

It is very difficult to grow up without the affection and love of your parents, whether through death or some other life tragedy that sends children into orphanages or the foster care system. However, it is a tragedy of our times—millions of young people growing up without parents. In Eastern Europe thousands have been orphaned because of war. In Africa the AIDS epidemic has wreaked similar havoc. Families have been separated as a result of war or natural disaster.

How sad it was to behold on the television screen parents separated from their children by Hurricane Katrina. Many children are yet missing. We are indeed living in perilous times (2 Timothy 3:1-5). Violence, war, and crime have indiscriminately killed millions of people in this century and separated many more. Others have been the victims of *'time and chance'*, like extreme poverty, which can befall anyone. (Ecclesiastes 9:11).

Unfortunately, many children have simply been abandoned by the ones given the responsibility to provide for them. Sadly, some parents have shown a shocking lack of 'natural affection' for their own progeny (2 Timothy 3:3). For others the abandonment is the end result of drug addiction, imprisonment, or alcoholism. Admittedly, there are also parents who abandon their children simply because of selfishness. Whatever the reason, being separated from one's parents is devastating.

These children may face a number of serious problems. Many government run foster care agencies have become little more than a readily available stockpile of already traumatized, vulnerable children, handed over to sexual predators – many times because the person's background was not thoroughly checked. A study conducted by the United Nations Children's Fund, called *Children in War,* reveals: "Unaccompanied children are the most vulnerable children—those who. . . face the harshest obstacles to survival, lack support for normal development and are abused. Separation from parents can be one of a child's most traumatic losses. They often fight *overwhelming* feelings of depression and frustration."

Exploitation and Murder of Children

In his book, *"Murder of the Innocents—Child-Killers and Their Victims"*, Paul Wilson states that "both the killers and the killed are caught up in a vicious cycle that society itself has created." It might seem strange to think that society may be responsible for, or at least may contribute to this tragedy, since most people find the exploitation of and the murder of children to be horrendous acts. Yet, industrialized societies, and even many less-developed ones, are saturated with films, TV productions, and reading material that glorify sex and violence.

There are now more and more hard-core pornographic films featuring children and even adults dressed up to resemble children. These depict explicit sex and violence involving children. Wilson further notes in his book that there are movie titles such as *Death of a Young One, Lingering Torture,* and *Dismembering for Beginners.* How large an audience do sadistic violence and pornography have? It is a *multibillion-dollar* industry!

Graphic violence and pornography have a tremendous impact on the lives of those who exploit children. A convicted sex offender who had murdered five young boys confessed: "I am a homosexual pedophile convicted of murder, and pornography was a determining factor in my downfall." Professor Berit Ås, of Oslo University, explains the effect child porn has: "We made a big mistake at the end of the 1960s. We believed that pornography could replace sex crimes by providing an outlet for sex offenders, and we took the lid off. Now we know we were wrong: such pornography *validates* sex crimes. It leads the offender to think, 'If I can watch this, it must be okay to do it.'" Watchtower, *"When Children Are Abducted by Strangers,"* 1995.

An adult's desire for titillation escalates as he becomes addicted to pornography. As a result, some are willing to use either coercion or violence to obtain children for their perverted use, including rape and murder.

Children Who Kill

Five carefully studied infant slayings in the Cleveland, Ohio area show that a preschool child is capable of murder. The victims, ranging in age from one and a half to eight months, had been dropped, bitten and beaten to death. Their assailants were children two to eight years old, apparently motivated by jealousy.

The parents of a young child found him in bed, his face discolored and swollen. An autopsy revealed that his skull had been fractured and part of his brain reduced to pulp. Of course, the parents were at first suspects but after careful investigation the police established that the murder was committed by two brothers living in a neighboring apartment. The small killers had dropped their victim repeatedly on the floor, struck him again and again with a woman's high-heeled shoe and bitten him several times. What was even more unusual, however, was the *age* of those involved: the murderers were only 5 and 2 years old...

A young child might be considered innocent by reason of its tender years. But actually, it would have to be a very young child to be considered innocent because of its years alone, for today we read of six-year-old murderers. One deliberately killed his father with a shotgun; another deliberately shot a playmate with a rifle. Such children pose problems for the police and the courts, as there is no legislation covering such youthful crimes—

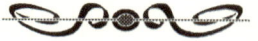

Source References

- A *Fact Sheet,* published by the National Committee for Prevention of Child Abuse (U.S.)
- Department of Health and Human Services (DHHS) (US), Administration on Children, Youth, and Families (ACF). Child maltreatment 2003 [online]. Washington (DC): Government Printing Office; 2005. [cited 2005 April 5].
- Department of Health and Human Services (DHHS), Administration on Children, Youth, and Families (ACF). Emerging practices in the prevention of child abuse and neglect. Washington (DC): Government Printing Office; 2003.
- Department of Health and Human Services (DHHS) (US), Administration on Children, Youth, and Families (ACF). In focus: understanding the effects of maltreatment on early brain development. Washington (DC): Government Printing Office; 2001.
- Felitti V, Anda R, Nordenberg D, Williamson D, Spitz A, Edwards V, et al. Relationship of childhood abuse and household dysfunction to many of the leading causes of death in adults. *American Journal of Preventive Medicine* 1998;14(4):245–58.
- Fromm S. Total estimated cost of child abuse and neglect in the United States — statistical evidence. Chicago (IL): Prevent Child Abuse America (PCAA); 2001. [cited 2005 Jan 1].
- National Center for Shaken Baby Syndrome website. [cited 2005 Jan 1]. Available from: URL: www.dontshake.com.
- Runyan D, Wattam C, Ikeda R, Hassan F, Ramiro L. Child abuse and neglect by parents and caregivers. In: Krug E, Dahlberg LL, Mercy JA, Zwi AB, Lozano R, editors. World Report on Violence and Health. Geneva, Switzerland: World Health Organization; 2002. p. 59-86.
- Tjaden P, Thoennes N. Full report of the prevalence, incidence, and consequences of violence against women: findings from the National Violence Against Women Survey. Washington (DC): National Institute of Justice; 2000 Nov. Report No.: NCJ 183721.

- BattleCry For a Generation, *"Youth Culture Crisis Guide"*
- Watchtower Bible and Tract Society of New York, Inc.
- Dr. Dale Conaway, *"Sex & The Bible"*, Destiny Image Publishers, Inc.
- Brennan Manning, *"The Ragamuffin Gospel"*
- National Association of Anorexia and Associated Disorders
- National Eating Disorders Association (NEDA)
- Eating Disorders Awareness and Prevention, Inc.
- American Association of Suicidology
- Joan Esherick, *"The Silent Cry"*, Mason Crest Publishers
- Essence Magazine, November Issue, 2005
- Watchtower, *"Watching The World"*
- Watchtower Bible and Tract Society of New York, Inc., *"Why Must I Live Without my Parents?"*
- TIME Magazine, *"Little Murderers"*
- New York *Times,* October 24, 1967; New York *Sunday News,* November 19, 1967.

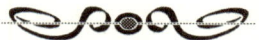

CHAPTER IV

THE CHALLENGE

"In The Beginning"…

The facts are irrefutable. **Promiscuity and perversion has created a culture that has swept the world, bringing about sad, violent, diseased death for its consequence**. Caught up in a society whose banner has been "do whatever feels good" and "believe whatever feels right", our civilization has experienced unprecedented spiritual and moral decay.

Man has attempted futilely and failed miserably in 'fixing' the world's problems – problems that *he created*. And the more he tries to fix, the 'broker' it gets. Man in his arrogance has been tampering with stuff that he had no business, like cloning animals (maybe somewhere, even *humans*…) He has created and unleashed *all kinds* of (un)natural disasters, creating suffering and massive loss of life: tsunamis, earthquakes, and so many hurricanes in 2005 that we ran out of names for them.

Even though the Earth brings forth enough food for the entire world, man's evil, selfish heart has created mass hunger, causing *millions* to go to bed (if they *have* one…) hungry. Man has caused mountains of ice and igloos to melt, producing floods. Mankind is instrumental in creating the destruction of the tropical rainforests, causing several of God's creatures to become extinct. An article in an October 2000 issue of the *Discover* magazine stated that **99% of all life that ever existed on this planet** – 99% of all animal, human, plant and marine life – **is now extinct**. We are left with a paltry *1%* of what was originally created – and are about to destroy that.

Man created *war* – murdering, raping, plundering, pilfering, burning, destroying more than life – but also *love* in the earth. Man has heedlessly continued on the destructive path, blaming God for his consequences. It is high time we begin to put the blame where it belongs – with *us*…

In a recent film, the character, Bruce, is frustrated with his 'nutty' job as a reporter who is assigned to a variety of inconsequential gigs. One night while driving home from work he begged God for a 'sign.' At that moment he saw to his left a flashing 'caution ahead' signal. Bruce ignored this warning, as a truck makes a turn in front of him – *loaded* with stop signs and other warning signals. Bruce is so busy complaining about the truck that in his attempt to pass it up, he doesn't notice the tree that he's about to crash his car into. So, with Bruce's car now crushed up and smoking the truck full of warning signs passes him by, while he swore and raved about life not being fair.

Bruce continued to try out for an anchor position being vacated by a 30-year veteran of the newscast but is bumped by an arrogant co-worker, who pokes fun at him at every turn. After discovering that he didn't get the job he wanted, Bruce publicly voices his sentiments on TV, loses his job and is thrown onto the street by his employers.

He lay there for a while and witnessed a group of young men taunting a disheveled, homeless man. Bruce attempted to stop them but is badly beaten, and is left lying in the street. He gathers what is left of his belongings, all the while screaming at and blaming God for his endless stream of misfortune.

To make a long story short, Bruce met 'god', who challenges him with the offer to take his place, 'since you think I'm doing such a poor job of answering prayers, son.' The conditions were that Bruce could do anything he wanted, except tamper with human will.

Well, Bruce played 'god' by 'parting' a bowl of soup and taking vengeance on the men who had beat him up. He went back to the TV station and by pulling strings, got the anchor job he wanted. To impress his girlfriend, Grace, he 'pulled' the moon closer, so he could romance her to vivid moonlight. (All during the picture I was wondering how 'Grace' could put up with such a moron. But she loved Bruce no matter what, constantly praying for him to 'find himself').

After awhile, though, Bruce found it difficult to keep up with the responsibilities of playing 'god' – and began looking for quick ways to fix problems -- responding to the millions of e-mailed prayers he received by answering 'yes' to all of them. This caused not only natural disasters (because of the moon situation, major floods erupted in various countries) but also economic problems (the stock market almost crashed). Also, the people who'd prayed to win the lottery (to which he replied 'yes' to *all*) were unhappy and started major rioting in the city, bringing it close to devastation.

In his callousness and increasing arrogance, Bruce's girlfriend caught him with the co-anchorwoman of the TV station. Grace ran out with Bruce close in tow behind, screaming that she couldn't leave him. And as she drove off, he yelled, "I'm the alpha. I'm the omega, baby... You can't leave *me*!" But she did... He tried to find 'god' – who by the way was doing the same thing he was doing when Bruce had first found him: mopping up a very large floor. As before, 'god' asked Bruce for his assistance in cleaning up the 'symbolic' mess he had made. As they mopped side by side, 'god' said to Bruce, "You know what is so fascinating? No matter, how filthy something gets, you can *always* clean it right up"...

Later, at his wits' end and after losing everything that ever really mattered in his life --including Grace -- Bruce stumbled out onto the street, and in the middle of torrential rain fell to his knees, sobbing. He threw up both hands and cried out, "Okay, God. I messed up, I messed up... You can have your job back. You know what's best for me. I give up.... I surrender to your will..."

The movie was thought-provoking and analogous. We ask God for signs and when He shows us 'blinking lights' and 'caution signals', 'slow down' warnings and 'stop' signs, we either don't recognize them or altogether ignore them. We're either too 'busy' to pay attention, too preoccupied with selfish desires, or too arrogant to *see* or *listen*.

"Be not deceived, God is not mocked. For whatsoever a man soweth, that shall he also reap. If you sow to the flesh you shall of the flesh reap corruption" (Galatians 6:7, 8) – God has already given us warning. Paraphrased it means 'don't be *tricked*, or take God lightly. His word is true and whatever He has spoken will surely come to pass.' God has said that certain 'actions' or 'deeds' we use our bodies, or *flesh*, to accomplish will 'produce a crop' (reap) of *corruption*. Words which also mean 'corruption': repulsiveness, foulness, repugnance, unpleasantness. In other words, *it's not good* -- but '*that*' is what we shall reap.

The crop is not going to come up *any different* than the *seeds* we plant (sow)... If we plant corn, *that* is what we'll get -- corn. If we plant beans, *that* is what we'll get. If we put some watermelon seeds down, don't be lookin' for *pineapples!* If we sow a wild, selfish, heedless, callous, vicarious life *that* is what we'll get: strange and bitter fruit.

Mankind has sown some *foul seeds* to the wind -- and is now reaping the *whirlwind*… We have tried so hard to be in control and play God without experience, understanding or qualifications. And as we have seen we're just no good at it. We've chosen on every hand to pursue our own selfish course and all we have proven is that we are weak and flawed – and independence from God has brought about nothing but *disaster*. It looks like we really messed this thing up, doesn't it? But is it too late? Is there hope? Where do we go from here? The answer resonates: *back to God*…

We should let the Loving One *who is* qualified for the job, have His job back….

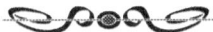

~ The Creator: "In The Beginning" ~

As a child growing up in the Church and a member of the Junior Choir, we used to sing, *"Somebody Bigger Than You and I."* Every time we sang the part about 'who writes the songs for the robins to sing and who hung the moon in the starry sky,' chills would run up and down my spine. I would cry because even in giddy youth I realized that everything in Creation was *designed*, carefully thought out and planned. The redbirds, bluebirds, yellow canaries all singing a different song, yet harmoniously, that I was awakened to happily every morning. The perfumed blossoms of many flowers flourishing in springtime, the rain falling when the earth is dry -- and only a *GREAT* Mind and a *HUGE* Being could be responsible...

Sir James Jeans, the British astronomer, said, "The universe appears to have been designed by a Pure Mathematician." As scientists muse over the precise order of the Earth, the solar system and entire stellar universe they acknowledge that 'the Master Planner left nothing to chance.' Former astronaut John Glenn noted "the orderliness of the whole universe about us," and that the galaxies were "all traveling in prescribed orbits in relation to one another." He therefore asked: "Could this have just *happened*? Was it an accident that a bunch of flotsam and jetsam suddenly started making these orbits of its own accord?" He concluded: "I can't believe that. . . . Some *Power* put all this into orbit and keeps it there."

It only takes a moment to gaze into the heavens and behold the moon and *zillions* of glittering stars, or feel the warmth of a glorious morning sunrise to know that there *must* be God somewhere. How do you account for the existence of lovely, living things, the various animals with bodies designed *ingenuously* to adapt to the habitat in which they live? Only a fantastically intelligent being could be responsible.

Regarding the mind-boggling precision of the universe, scholars and scientists have concluded that the slant of the Earth at an angle of 23 degrees produces seasons. They say if the Earth had not been tilted as it is, vapors from the oceans would move both north and south, piling up entire *continents* of ice. If the moon were only 50,000 miles away from Earth instead of 200,000, the tides might be so enormous that all continents would be submerged under water. If the Earth's crust had been only 10 feet thicker, there would be no oxygen, which without it all animal life would die. Though the Earth's weight is estimated at six sextillion tons (a six with *21 zeros*, people...), it is perfectly balanced and turns easily on its axis. All throughout Creation, there is an apparent Magnificent Power revealed that bewilders us, *captivates* and should enamor us to this God of obvious and *enormous* love.

As a great artist who draws on canvas, whose work is highly recognized and cannot be attributed to another, so is God's divine signature present on *all* His handiwork. Looking at the spectacular approach He utilized -- the canvas of the universe -- to exhibit His Masterful creation, there can be only one artist responsible for it. This is the deduction expressed by one Bible writer who said regarding the physical heavens: *"Lift up your eyes on high, and behold. Who has created these things? It is the One who is bringing forth the army of them even by number, all of whom he calls even by name."* It is the' One' *that created the heavens, and stretched them out; he that spread forth the earth; he that gives breath to the people upon it and spirit to them that walk therein."* —Isaiah 40:26; 42:5.

Such a sense of awe and reverence is instilled as I consider the absolute greatness and sovereignty of God, and when I read Psalms 90:1, 2 in the Holy Writ: *"Lord, thou hast been my dwelling place in all generations. Before the mountains were brought forth, or ever thou hast formed the earth and the world, even from everlasting to everlasting, thou art God."* This verse speaks of the origin of Our Creator. *From* eternal infinity *to* eternal infinity, God has always existed and has no beginning and no ending.

Before time *was* 'time' and before 'space' had a name, God was preexistent, bringing all things into being. Cosmologists, evolutionists and other scientists say the earth, galaxies and stars are billions of years old. However, they will never know the age of the earth. Man's devices of time measurement are inadequate in relation to God. *"For as the heavens are higher than the earth, so are my thoughts higher than your thoughts"* (Isaiah 55:9). Scientific knowledge is frustrated from wondering what puzzling power is holding it all together. But unless one honestly seeks an experience with God, he cannot understand these things.

No "big boom" is responsible for the beautiful, orderly fashion that the earth spins on its axis, or the way the brilliant sun rotates without catching everything on fire, or without colliding into another bright star and *somehow* we're not flung callously spinning in the darkness. Everything is much too precise, too systematic and too balanced to dismiss to haphazard chance. The universe is too intricately coordinated to relegate its existence to the explosion of gases.

The Bible tells us who is responsible:

God looked into the void of the farthest reaches of the stratosphere and saw a little dark corner, got an idea and declared, *"I think I'll make me a world."* *God stepped* out onto nothing and declared, *"Let there be Light",* and light shot from *somewhere* out of the darkness; He called the light "Day" and the darkness "Night." *God took* the dry land and separated it from the waters and said, *"The dry land is 'Earth',"* and then gathered together the waters and called them 'Seas'. God declared, *"Let the earth bring forth grass, the herb yielding seed and fruit after every kind",* and it would be so. He declared, *"Let there be lights in the firmament of the heaven, and let them be for signs and for seasons, for days and years."*

"And God made two great lights; the greater light to rule the day (the Sun), and the lesser light to rule the night (the Moon): he made the stars also." And God said, *"Let the waters bring forth abundantly the moving creatures that hath life, and birds that may fly above the earth in the open firmament of heaven. And God created great whales, and every living creature that moves."* And God saw that it was good... (Genesis 1:121)*

We cannot get around it. No matter how hard we try the facts yet point to this: Superb organization requires a superb organizer. Nothing in our experience indicates that anything organized happens by *chance*, by *accident*. Rather, our entire experience in life shows that everything organized must have an organizer. Every man-made machine, car, computer, or building had a maker, a designer, an architect, an organizer – someone who could logically put the pieces together. So rationally, the far more complex and inconceivable organization that exist in the universe must have had an organizer, too. Such immense size, meticulousness and law as exist throughout the universe could never have happened just by *accident.* All these things *must* be the products of a Superior Mind.

His name is "*YeHoWaH*" ('*Jehovah*', in Latin), which means "He Who Causes To Become." The Divine Purposer is renown for his exploits. *"I am the Lord... new things I declare: before they spring forth I tell you of them"* (Isaiah 42:8, 9). *"I am God... Declaring the end from the beginning and from ancient times the things that are not yet done"* (Isaiah 46:9, 10).

God's unique name serves to differentiate Him from all other gods. His name, *YHWH*, appears more than 7,000 times in the Hebrew text of the Old and New Testament Scriptures. However, over the course of centuries, the correct pronunciation of *YHWH* was lost. Jewish scholars in the Middle Ages developed a system of symbols placed beneath and beside the consonants (the *Tetragrammaton*) to indicate the missing vowels ('*YaHoWeH'*). The word so often substituted in the Holy Scriptures for the divine name is 'Adonai', or 'LORD' and is an enigma.

YHWH is God's most common Hebrew name found more than 6,000 times in the Old Testament. Reverence for the divine name led to the practice of avoiding its use lest one should break the Third Commandment (Exodus 20:7 – *"You shall not use the name of your God in vain...For the LORD will not hold him guiltless that does"*).

Israel had a great reverence for God's name, perhaps because the Mosaic Law taught that those who disrespected the name of God would be put to death (Leviticus 24:16). In time it was thought that the divine name was too holy to pronounce at all. The name of God was so sacred to the ancient Jewish scribes that they began the practice of writing the divine name with a special pen, solely used for this purpose. After saying a prayer, they would write God's name with the designated pen. And which after writing the divine name would pick up the regular pen and resume their work.

Yes, God's name is significant and an important key in disclosing His doctrine, character, power, holiness and desired relationship with His people. And based upon the various aspects of God and each biblical character's personal encounter or relationship with Him, other names were ascribed to Him:

- **El-Shaddai** (Genesis 17:1-2), which means "Almighty God"
- **El-Elyon** (Numbers 24:16), which means "Most High God" or "Exalted One"
- **El-Olam** (Psalm 90:2), which means "God of Eternity," or "God, the Everlasting One"
- **El-Berith** (2 Corinthians 34:32), which means "God Who Sees Me" or "God of Vision"
- **Elohim,** a plural form of deity, is used in Genesis 1:26 where the Bible says, "And God said, *'Let us make man in our image, after our likeness.'*

The Lord's name has been the subject of discussion for thousands of years. However, our Heavenly Father is primarily concerned with whether or not we know *Him* in his relationship to humankind, and not with the *pronunciation* of His name. An earthly father doesn't become angry when his young child just learning to talk says, "Da-Da" instead of "Daddy". A good father will be *thrilled* that his child is beginning to recognize him as father. God is happy when we realize His *role* in our lives – Father and Creator – and His *goal*: to be *recognized* and *acknowledged* as such by His human creation. The most wonderful reality of God is that He is Father to us *all* – because He created us all…

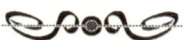

~ The Creation: "What Is Man?" ~

"What is man that thou art mindful of him, or the son of man that thou visiteth him?"

I have often sat in reflection, pondering the concept of God *stooped* beside a clear body of water, mixing water with dirt, *designing* what would be the masterpiece of His perfect Creation: Man. God looked around and saw that everything He had made to this point was not only good, but *very* good… But *this* was to be the crowning glory of all Creation. He had taken a 'short-cut' on some of Creation – like *speaking* Light, the fowl and sea life into existence. But Jehovah opted to take a hands-on approach for this special project, engaging all of His divine abilities: concentration, inspiration, imagination, time, patience, gentleness, great care, interest, consideration and anticipation. The very thought of it prompted King David to ask: *"When I study your heavens, the work of your fingers, the moon and stars, which you have ordained;* what is man, *that you are attentive to him? And the son of man, that you go to him?"* (Psalms 8:3, 4)

The emotion God used above all to create this being was *LOVE*… With His GOD capacity for love He molded this lump of clay into His own resemblance and divine likeness, and *"blew the breath of life into man's nostrils and 'man' became a living soul* (Genesis 2:7). After breathing eternity into man, God placed the first human, 'Adam', in the environs of Edenic paradise, with the prospect that man would live forever on earth. After assigning Adam the duty of naming *'every living creature'*, God in loving concern discovered *there was not found an help meet* for Adam (Genesis 2:20).

And the Lord caused a deep sleep to fall upon Adam…and he took one of his ribs and closed up the flesh. And the rib God had taken from man, made He a woman, and brought her unto the man (Genesis 2:21, 22). *And God blessed them and said, "Be fruitful and multiply, populate and have dominion over everything upon the earth. And God saw everything that He had made, and it was very good. It was the sixth day* (Genesis 1:28-31).

~~~~~~~~~~~~~~~~~~~~

The rather simplistic depiction of man's creation on the previous page is in harmony with scientific truth. All the elements of which the human body is composed are to be found in the "dust from the ground." A chemist once claimed that an adult human body is 65 percent oxygen, 18 percent carbon, 10 percent hydrogen, 3 percent nitrogen, 1.5 percent calcium, and 1 percent phosphorus, with the remainder being made up of other elements. Whether these estimates are wholly accurate is unimportant. The fact remains: We are *dust*...

Who apart from *God* could create such elaborate creatures out of nothing more than dust? God's works are perfect and without flaw, so His choosing to create man in this way is certainly no cause for criticism. That the divine Creator was able to create man from the dust of the earth in an awe-inspiring and wonderful way should increase our appreciation of His vast love, power and wisdom.—Deuteronomy 32:4, Psalm 139:14.

The oldest written record of human history, the Bible, informs us that our first parents enjoyed perfection and had the prospect of seeing the whole earth become a glorious paradise occupied by perfect humans, living in lasting peace and happiness. That was God's purpose in creating the earth and mankind. However, creatures of dust have limitations...

Adam and Eve disobeyed God and brought about a horribly changed situation for their entire future human family. Being made of dust then took on new connotations. No longer *perfect*, mankind became damaged goods, 'flawed flesh' which was in hostile opposition to a holy God, who is a *Spirit* (St. John 4:24). Through their disobedience, Adam and Eve proved that their desire was no longer towards God. *"For the desires of the flesh struggle against the Spirit, and the Spirit against the flesh: and these are contrary the one to the other: so that you cannot do that which is right"* (Galatians 5:17).

In other words, as a result of our First Parents' original sin, every human since born was imperfect – with inherited AIDS, our own *personal* 'Acquired Immune DeficiencieS'. Hence, the reason babies are born with missing limbs/body parts, the reason some are born with multiples of limbs/body parts, the reason a young child can die from cancer, the reason some are born with male *and* female genitalia, the reason some are born female in a male's body and vice versa, the reason hate, murder and sexual deviance is often manifested in *kids*. *Stop arguing* as to what aberration cannot be manifested in human flesh! The Word clearly states *'there is no good thing that the flesh is capable of.'* There should be *no* question, *no* confusion as to the multiplicity of defects that the flesh is capable of producing. Too much precious time is wasted dealing with the symptoms rather than the cure. If we treat the 'terminal cancer' of sin, the subsequent symptoms of sin will no longer be manifested.

The Honorable Minister Louis Farrakhan profoundly stated in a 1992 sermon, "Adam brought death because he brought rebellion, causing us to live from the navel down… Adam *fell*. He didn't fall from the Empire State Building. He fell from a state of mind that made him one with his Creator. Adam's fall sentenced human kind to death: physical death, in that we live so short a time, but the greatest death of all is *spiritual* death, because we have become estranged from Allah (God)…

Had Adam and Eve remained faithful to God, they would never have erred, sinned, so as to become flawed, or need forgiveness. Nor would they (or we) have ever experienced suffering of any kind. Above all, they would never have had to die, or descend into the dark abyss of spiritual separation from the Creator, whereby we would need redemption…

~~~~~~~~~~~~~~~~~

I am sure we all saw and were rapt by the *magnificent* and -- by Mel Gibson's own admission -- Holy Ghost-inspired work of "Passion of the Christ". It was so amazing that I saw it twice, reaffirming my belief in the Lord. Who would have ever imagined that the big screen would one day extend such a *powerful* altar call? For though some read and understand what the scriptures say about the ransom sacrifice of Christ for the sins of mankind, some others need *pictures*. So breathtakingly *real* was The Passion's portrayal, that *murderers* who had never been caught and had gotten away scot-free, saw the movie, admitted the crime, turned themselves into authorities and confessed belief in Christ's sacrifice.

"For God so loved the world that He gave His only begotten Son; that whosoever believeth in Him should not perish: but have everlasting life. God sent not His Son to condemn the world, but so that all through Him might be saved" (St. John 3:16, 17) Yes, Jesus Christ paid the ransom price necessary to retrieve mankind's lost heritage and get us back in right relationship with God. The word 'ransom' signifies the sum paid to redeem a captive and denotes 'equivalency'. It was *at* a tree *in* a Garden that man lost his perfection and identity as a son of God. But it was in another Garden (Gethsemane) and *on* a tree that Jesus the Christ paid a *great* price to obtain mankind's identity back as sons of God.

Only a perfect human life could be the equivalent of what Adam lost. Therefore, Jesus is referred to in the New Testament as 'the second Adam'. Since death came by the first created, *human* son of God (Adam), eternal life came through Jesus Christ -- the perfect, first created (or *'first begotten'*) *Spirit* son of God. Since you can only have one first of *anything*, Jesus Christ was the *first created being* by Jehovah God. Hence, Jesus was 'in the beginning' with God and all other things were made by Him, along with His Father. *"The same was in the beginning with God; all things were made by Him..."* (St. John 1:2).

According to the Bible, every being created by God is referred to as a 'son': angels, the devil, who had been an angel, are created *spirit* sons of God. *"Again there was a day when the sons of God came to present themselves before the Lord, and Satan came...to present himself also"* (Job 2:1) However, when Satan caused war in heaven by attempting to usurp God's authority and was banished, he took *one-third* of the angels with him. *"And there was war in heaven: Michael and his angels fought against the dragon. The dragon fought along with his angels but did not prevail. And the great dragon was cast out, that old serpent called the Devil and Satan, which deceived the whole world: he was cast out into the earth and his angels were cast out with him."* (Revelation 12:7, 8 & 9). *"Woe to the inhabitants of the earth and the sea! For the devil has come down unto you, having great rage because he knows he has but a short time"* (Revelation 12:12).

Listening to the Deceiver was why mankind lost his inheritance in the Garden of Eden – Now *he's here* on earth, trying hard to cause man to lose his inheritance once again -- but this time *eternally*…

We wrestle not against flesh and blood but against spiritual powers, against principalities… Weak, faltering and flawed in nature, we alone cannot handle such an all-out, no-holds barred, vicious, spiritual assault. Mankind has been *pummeled*, enduring the bitter consequences of our First Parents disobedience…

~~~~~~~~~~~~~~~~~

After it became necessary to put Adam and Eve out of the Garden of Eden, God agonized over His decision. He had first cursed the serpent for deceiving the couple. *"Because you have done this, upon your belly shall you go, dust shall you eat all your days. I will put enmity between you and woman. Her seed shall bruise your head, and you shall bruise his heel."* To Eve, God said: *"I will greatly multiply your sorrow and your conception; in sorrow shall you bring forth children; and your desire shall be to your husband, who shall rule over you."* He had cursed man to till the soil. *"In the sweat of your face shall you eat bread, till you return to the ground; for out of it were you taken. Dust you are and unto dust shall you return"* (Genesis 3:17-19). Had God allowed Adam and Eve to remain in the Garden they would have partook of the tree of life, and lived forever in disobedience.

No, He had done the right thing. And even though God knew what the couple's choice would be it yet broke His heart. God was distressed over His now flawed human creation because He knew what would be the consequences of their sin: pain, suffering, agony, violence, sorrow, grief, disappointment, rejection, loss, hunger, temptation, lust, greed, the defect of imperfection, disease – and *death*… He knew that Adam and Eve's human bodies would be ravaged by attempting to appease their now predominant quality, the *flesh*. He imagined a disease called 'AIDS' which would come about largely due to sexual transgression, and knew that He had not designed the human body to withstand such abuses…

The human body was created, designed and planned to interconnect and experience spiritual communion with God. The Great Creator fashioned man quite uniquely from any other creature, endowing him with certain God-like qualities. **Man's structure is comprised of both body (flesh) and spirit:** the breath of God that imparted *animation*, *conscience* (which embodies the power of free choice), *intellect* and *emotion* to man. *"And the Lord God formed man from the dust of the earth, and breathed into his nostrils the breath of life and <u>man</u> <u>became</u> a <u>living soul</u>"* (Genesis 2:7).

Man's structure consists of three major components: body (flesh), mind (spiritual) and spirit, the chief component. These components serve as conduits, or channels, one into the other. For instance, whatever is channeled into the **body** via the five senses is passed on to the **mind**, which processes it and passes it along to the **spirit**. **The true spirit of man can only be revealed by his actions.** In other words, man 'acts out' whatever has been internalized. If a person's actions are good, then it stands to reason he has internalized only pleasant things. However, in the reverse, evil actions are a result of evil ingestion. The ruling entity of the body and spirit is the mind, which is a spiritual component. It is controlled by either good or evil, depending solely on what is taken into the body via the senses.

In order to function as whole, healthy beings, we need to see how God intended for humans to function – *including* within the context of sexuality. **Sexual intercourse is more than just a *physical* act but is also a door into the *spirit* realm.** The Bible has always attached spiritual import to this act, as **you cannot be united sexually without involving the most essential part of your human construction: your *spirit*.** Sexual intercourse is a covenantal, divine endowment that impacts us at the very core of our being -- a *spiritual act* that is governed by *spiritual laws*. Human sexuality must be understood within the context of its spiritual foundation. Failure to view it thusly has resulted in personal frustration and societal decay, as we have seen. **<u>When spiritual laws are broken, spiritual penalties are enforced</u>**. Dr. Dale H. Conaway, *"Sex & The Bible: A Biblical Perspective of Human Sexuality,"* 1996.

When Paul stated in 1 Corinthians 6:13b, *"The body is not for fornication"*, it was not a self-righteous, pious declaration. The statement had spiritual, physiological and medical implications. The Greek word translated "fornication" is *por·nei´a* and embodies every form of human sexual immorality and deviance: homosexuality, unlawful heterosexual intercourse (rape or sex outside of marriage), beastiality and prostitution. *Porneia* is understood to involve the grossly immoral use of the genital organ(s) of at least one human; also there must have been two or more parties (including another consenting human or a beast), whether of the same sex or the opposite sex. I am sure you also notice and understand the implication of the prefix *'porn'*. Paul's statement to the hedonistic Epicureans of his day gave clarity to the human sexual dilemma: *the human body was simply not fashioned or equipped to endure the ravages of sexual sin...*

~~~~~~~~~~~~~~~~~

For the sake of clarity, let us veer briefly from the intellectual to the more inane, shall we? The following analogies are given to provide some idea as to how God must feel when we use and abuse our beautiful and *amazingly* crafted bodies, engaging in sexual sin:

A clothes designer has made a simply fantastic line of exclusive dresses for smaller framed women, sizes 2 to 8. One day, she happens to see one of her designs – on a *300-pound woman*! Of course, the designer is disturbed because her beautiful, creative design -- which is a reflection of her -- has been misused. And on a 300-pounder, her design is misshapen and bears no resemblance to her original creation or intent.

Our predicament is also much like an engineer who designs and builds a special car – and it's a *lean, mean* drivin' machine. The engineer gives much time and attention to detail in building this car, as his intention is to enter it in the Biggest Race. He knows how much force and pressure the car can take, how fast it will go without busting any gaskets, cams or valves, where every bolt, screw and optional feature will be and exactly who he wants to *drive* the car -- himself. Let's say that when the car is completed the engineer puts it in pristine surroundings – perhaps on a showroom floor. However, *another* engineer who has watched the entire creation of the car and saw the care and attention given it, becomes *jealous*. He feels the car should belong to *him*, for whatever reason, and decides to sabotage the car. Racing it at a speed excessive to its design, a couple of gaskets blew in the engine and some screws came out. The second engineer sneakily places the damaged car back in the showroom. However, when the engineer who designed and built the car saw the dirty tires, screws in places they didn't belong and smoking engine, he knew immediately who was at fault. He also knew the car would have to be withdrawn from the race, as it was damaged, *flawed* and no longer in perfect condition...

Even though the two parallels given in *no way* compare to the love and *consideration* that God put into the creation of the human body, hopefully you get the point. The point being: we have been applying too much force, going *too fast* and using our 'car' for things it never was designed to withstand. We have been inflicting serious damage to certain essential *parts* of our 'car'. Lastly, we are sticking 'screws' in places they were *never* intended to go...

~~~~~~~~~~~~~~~~~~~

Sinful lusts are those things we desire that are forbidden by God. The desire for intimacy in itself is not sinful, as God placed that 'feature' in us. However, our desires become sinful when we seek to fulfill them against God's Word. As stated earlier, it is impossible to be united sexually without involving your *spirit*. So then if we join to a person in fornication, adultery or sexual sin against the Word of God, we are actually joining ourselves to an 'evil' spirit. Thus, an *ungodly* soul tie can develop and bind us to dangerous people and habits. These ties feed on lust, idolatry, covetousness, witchcraft and sexual sin. Dr. Dale H. Conaway, *"Sex & The Bible: A Biblical Perspective of Human Sexuality,"* 1996.

When we engage our bodies in sexual activities, a dynamic takes place in us that result in a type of emotional and psychological dependence. This *dependency* is directed to whomever we yield our body to – even if it is a one-night stand... *"What? Know you not that he which is joined to an harlot is one body? For two, saith He, shall be one flesh"* (1 Corinthians 6:16). *"Know you not that to whom you yield yourselves, you become a slave to obey?"* (Romans 6:16).

Ungodly soul ties that develop as a result of sexual sin are *extremely* difficult to break, binding one emotionally, spiritually and physically, and are often mistaken for true love. These ties produce spiritual *bondage*, pain, dependence, confusion and misery – and in many cases, *other* negative practices and addictions. I know there are some who may have either experienced themselves or know of someone in an abusive situation, who simply could not walk away. Some people, particularly women, have become hooked on drugs, turned to prostitution or *killed* simply because they wouldn't leave an abusive relationship. In many of these instances, an ungodly soul tie of total dependence had been formed. This is one reason why sexual sin is so dangerous; it brings about destructive consequences...

But what is a *soul tie*? It is the emotional, psychological and physiological dependence an individual develops toward another person or thing. It is the captivation of one's mind and emotions, and it is formed when one yields his body to a person or thing (Romans 6:12-16). The most acceptable soul tie is God-ordained and develops in the context of marital intimacy. In marriage the spirit is engaged with the true entity and sex is sanctioned and hallowed. The human body is the 'temple' of the Holy Spirit. True worship involves yielding the body in surrender to the object of worship. The unification and communion that is experienced in holy matrimony is what God intended in His relationship to mankind – to be the object of total yielding of body, mind and spirit *in worship.*

When God performed the first human marriage he said: *"...a man will leave his father and his mother and cleave to his wife, and they will become one flesh."* (Genesis 2:24). Here the standard set for man and woman was monogamy, and promiscuous sexual behavior was ruled out. Also, no consideration for divorce and remarriage was given.

Jehovah did not form Eve from the dust as He had Adam because He wanted man and woman to share a unique intimacy. In giving Eve a part of Adam (a rib taken from his side), God created a complete bonding of the physical, emotional and spiritual -- eternally uniting the couple. Not only was there a transfer of Adam's flesh, but of bone, which produces blood. The life of all flesh is in the blood. Dr. Dale H. Conaway, *"Sex & The Bible: A Biblical Perspective of Human Sexuality,"* 1996.

Physical prostration of the body implies rendering, yielding and submitting. Sexual intercourse is the ultimate form of 'giving' your total being—mind, spirit and body -- to a person. When we engage in sexual intercourse, we are joining to unseen spiritual forces -- constituting spiritual identification and attachment. In the perverting of human sexuality, sex becomes an object of false worship and a source of demonic defilement. *"Sex &The Bible: A Biblical Perspective of Human Sexuality,"* 1996.

In breaking ungodly soul ties several key elements are involved: repentance (or forsaking this relationship), and accepting God's salvation. If ungodly soul ties are not confessed, forsaken and *healed*, it will produce recurring detriment to you, your other interpersonal relationships and later, your offspring. At all costs, ungodly soul ties should be *completely severed* if one is to break free from the past – and go on to establish a true and *Godly* soul connection…

~~~~~~~~~~~~~~~~~~

Perhaps the most unfortunate thing that has been done by modern religion is the part it has played in reducing God in the opinion of the world to a small-minded, capricious, austere, eternal note taker, who uses indelible ink. Not a *drop* of love or compassion in him. This ludicrous, conjured image of someone's not-so-sane imagination, possesses not a modicum of warmth, is aloof, and is *always* on the ready to chronicle your many offences in dusty ledgers, punish you and *can't wait* to send you to hell. So as soon as you *die* your carcass will be condemned, sentenced *before* you are judged, sent to eternal 'life' (not *death,* 'cause if you're *dead* you wouldn't be able to weep *or* knash your teeth…) in hell. Then when Judgment Day comes at the end of the world, somehow you're hauled up from hell again to be judged, condemned, sentenced – the whole thing starts all over again…

From listening to some people's concept of God, one would get the notion that he was identical to the 'great and powerful Wizard of Oz.' As we remember from youth, The Wizard would summon pitiable, quaking-in-their-boots individuals into his presence, slap-happy over the way the pathetic, menial earthlings responded to his booming voice and lowering appearance. He would ask these inconsequential creatures what they wanted, with roaring flames leaping behind him -- all the while knowing he was powerless to fulfill any of their desires, sending them on wild goose chases.

Proclaimers of 'gloom and doom' range from super scary legalists who *prefer* a God of justice and wrath, to the timid, cautious, tip-toer around the embracing love of God, as if it were a poisonous adder waiting to strike at the least hint of acceptance. The face of a compassionate God has been concealed. How unfortunate it is that we have such a *hard time* accepting that God is Love, as revealed through His son, Christ Jesus, but have absolutely no problem embracing the God of Judgment. How is it that we can wrap our minds around the most far-fetched, *ludicrous,* illogical man-invented stuff but when it comes to God, we suddenly have some kind of *brain* burp ('Sorry, information does not register-does not register-does not register'...) Have we been hurt so bad that it is just *too* inconceivable to believe that someone so GREAT can love the *mess* out of us? Well, *God does...*

Everything God is, *is for us.* Everything God *does* is *for us*: the breathtaking beauty of His created world, the thoughtful care that went into its planning. God's love-filled fashioning of man in His own image from the dust of the earth was only surpassed by the kiss of Life that He planted on the lips of His human creation. God made us so that every microscopic, miniscule, part of our body serves a vital purpose. Our *eyelashes*, as inconsequential as they seem to be, protect our very vision. God knows us so intimately that even the number of hairs on each head, He knows.

He knows what delights, frights, frustrates, tempts, disappoints, hurts, angers, saddens, violates and abuses us. He knows our thoughts afar off, our strengths, weaknesses, incapacities, deficiencies, accomplishments, failures, likes, loves, dislikes and various intricacies. God knows us *intrinsically* -- and is concerned about everything that concerns us. But not only is God concerned about us. He is absolutely, positively, undeniably, *crazy* in love with us! God *is* Love...

Remember that movie I was telling you about – about Bruce and his girlfriend, Grace? Though Bruce was a silly, arrogant, selfish, irresponsible, defiant, sanctimonious imbecile, Grace accepted him fully, just as he was. Though Bruce constantly took her for granted, fooled around on her and disappointed her at every turn, she still loved and *prayed* for him.

Well, God's grace does so much more. Even though we have all sinned and fallen short of His glory, He loves us right on. God hurts when we hurt, even though we've been the ones hurting ourselves through disobedience to Him. Still, as Brennan Manning stated, God has one, solitary, unrelenting attitude toward mankind: He *loves* us. But of course this is too incredible to comprehend – especially for those huffing and puffing to impress God by pulling themselves up by their own bootstraps. The concept of grace is impossible to grasp for those scrambling to earn a merit badge for good deeds done.

Grace is a *gift*. If someone says, "I have a gift for you," you know exactly what that means: it's *free*!!! You're to be given something 'of great price' from someone who apparently cares an awful lot about you that you don't have to work for, nor pay for – nor, in fact, *deserve*.   It is a *gift* – and the only thing that is expected of you is that you *accept* the gift. *"By grace are you saved, through faith; not because of your own merits, but it is a gift of God. Grace is not earned by your good deeds, lest you should have something to brag about"* (Ephesians 2:8, 9 paraphrased)

Through no merit of our own, but *solely* by His mercy we have been restored to a right relationship with God through our acceptance of the life, death and resurrection of His beloved Son, Jesus Christ. Thomas Merton stated, "A saint is not someone who is good but who experiences the goodness of God."

There is only one requirement by which we have access to this grace: Jesus said, *"Truly I say to you, Whoever shall not receive the kingdom of God as a child shall in no way enter into it"* (St. Luke 18:17). The major point emphasized here is that there is *nothing* we can do in and of ourselves to inherit the Kingdom: no good deeds, no earning brownie points and no extra credit assignments. We must simply receive grace as 'little children'.

What is it about 'little children' that God loves? Well, for one thing children haven't *done* anything. They have no past, no heavy baggage to shuffle from place to place. They are not encumbered with guilt, nor are they scrambling to impress. They live in the present, content with whatever you provide for them and they are too small to fret about the future. So, in essence children know *nothing*. And we should all just *rush* out and get our hands on one of those 'Little Children' templates because *that's* what God wants. He doesn't need another know-it-all, finger-pointing, chest-smoter incensing Him with smug, sanctimonious droning about good works, kept laws, straight walks, prayed prayers, tithe-paying, alms-giving, Sunday sacraments, da-da-da... For all our showboating and professed rightness, it means *nothing* to God. *"But we are all as an unclean thing, and all our righteousnesses are as filthy rags"* (Isaiah 64:6). We must come before God *relying solely* on His grace and mercy.

In his emotive book, *"The Ragamuffin Gospel,"* the brilliant, *hilarious* Brennan Manning relates a story concerning the essence of child-like acceptance of grace. He wrote about how a little three-year old came to his home with his parents. "I looked down and said, 'Hi, John. I am delighted to see you.' Little John looked neither to the right nor left. His face was set like flint. With the apocalyptic glint of an aimed gun, he narrowed his eyes and demanded, 'Where's the cookies?' The Kingdom belongs to people who aren't trying to look good or impress anybody, even themselves. All he has to do is happily accept the 'cookies' – the *hand-out* of the free grace of God."

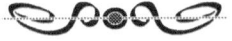

In its World AIDS Day statement, the Vatican's department on health issues blamed the spread of HIV on "the pansexual culture that devalues sexuality, reducing it to a mere pleasure without further significance." The church holds that promoting the use of condoms fosters lifestyles and behavior that will spread the virus.

The pope calls recent AIDS statistics "alarming," and he praises church efforts to help those infected. "I encourage the many initiatives being promoted to eliminate this disease," he says. "I feel close to those sick with AIDS and their families and I invoke for them the help and comfort of the Lord," Pope Benedict XVI says in a message issued for World AIDS Day. The pontiff avoids, however, the controversial matter of the Roman Catholic Church's opposition to the use of condoms.

The church opposes condoms, except in rare circumstances, because they are a form of contraception. A case in which an HIV-positive man insists on having sex with his wife is sometimes cited by church experts as an example of such an exception.

[This summary provided by the CDC National Center for HIV, STD, and TB Prevention | Reuters | November 30, 2005 | Philip Pullella]

~~~~~~~~~~~~~~~~

As previously stated, whenever "the Church" is mentioned in this book, it is a reference to a 'community of like-minded people.' Also, I for my part do not wish to infer specific racial or denominational designations, e.g., black, white, Hispanic, etc. when addressing the church. Because on the issue of AIDS it appears that most churches are stuck in the belief that HIV/AIDS is a 'gay disease' that cannot possibly exist among their flock. Others who *know* of the disease, refuse to address it and apparently think that if they ignore it long enough, the disease will somehow go away.

For the most part, the Church as a viable community organization has refused to address the HIV/AIDS issue in an effective, concerted manner. The disproportionately few pastors who are educated on the subject and dare to broach it tend to disagree over acceptable ways to educate – whether to advocate safer-sex, or preach total abstinence. While gathering information from a few pastors to include in this book, I was told: "What can be said about this? You really can't tell people not to have sex…"

The Reverend Roderick Hennings, a pastor in Buffalo, New York, has no desire to protest the inclusion of safer-sex information in *other* people's workshops. However, he is clear that it is not something he believes the church should do. "Public health officials advocate condoms and spermicides, and I'm not against that public policy," he says, "but there is another level of morality and policy that is ecclesiastically based. Regardless of the standards of the secular world, we still have to preach what is right" (+hivplus Magazine, *"The Enlightenment"*, February 2004, hivplusmag.com).

One thing is abundantly clear, however. As HIV continues to spread rampantly among Blacks, it has become of utmost urgency that the church establishes some form of dialogue and policy in educating their congregants and fighting this pandemic. It is *essential* that the church establish educational opportunities on a national level, to be equipped with language and knowledge to address sexuality issues for teens, their parents and/or guardians. The legacy of silence from the pulpit about sexual issues has had a tremendous negative impact on the community. It's time to break the silence…

On the following pages, you will be introduced to modern-day bishops, pastors and ministers who have their finger on the pulse of the community and society at large. I sought out the counsel of these spiritual leaders, who are broad in their scope of ministry and ever effectively addressing every spiritual, physical and emotional need of humankind.

These men and women are knowledgeable and educated of the times in which we live, having been tried in the fire of 'people' ministry in their churches, on the streets, in homeless shelters and prisons. They have continually assisted in every way -- feeding, clothing, caring for, nursing, providing shelter and spiritual instruction to this city's most hapless victims and disenfranchised:

- Pastor Charles Roach has given *profound* spiritual teaching and instruction to St. Louis' pastors and ministers, has a vibrant men's ministry and has ministered over 25 years at the Harbor Light Mission; vibrant youth ministry
- Minister Samson Latchison has a vital ministry dealing with psychotic youth in his city; has ministered in Guatemala and South Africa, building homes and classrooms
- Archbishop Michael A. West, Sr. in *deep* ministry that has existed nearly half a century; spiritual instructor to most in *all* areas of ministry, including bishopric. Operates a food pantry wherein people receive items that rival shopping at upscale markets: Loreal shampoo, Bayer aspirin, Tyson chicken breasts. For 20 years of Thanksgivings, **100** families receive *groceries*, which includes a 12 pound turkey and much more
- Caring Reverend Larry Rice almost *single-handedly* provides for St. Louis' entire homeless community, which is a Herculean effort of mammoth proportion. Has slept outside in a cardboard box, in bitterly cold St. Louis temps to draw attention to the plight of the homeless
- Dynamic Bishop George White, Jr. simultaneously pastors two large churches; has most effective prison, alcohol/drug rehab and AIDS church ministries in the area. Feeds homeless every Sunday morning; vibrant youth ministry
- Bishop Dr. Wyatt I. Greenlee, Jr., an effective pastor that ministers strictly 'out-of-the-box' and reaches where you are; many local, national and international affiliations; *awesome* church music ministry and outreach ministry
- Evangelist Ruth Latchison Nichols, a compassionate lover of youth. Founded in 1992 vital youth ministry, targeting the underachiever – conducting self-esteem workshops, parenting skills, etc. Dynamic prison and nursing home ministries
- Dr. Ralph Petty, a powerful pastor in the area whose message of God's grace has saved countless lives. Ministry of compassion to AIDS victims – and to all of us that need hope; *dynamic* outreach ministry to the infirmed and choir ministry
- Reverend Carl Smith, Sr., a capable pastor with the heart and ability to deal with troubled youth. Founder of "Operation

Safe Haven", a vibrant youth, after-school ministry aimed at keeping children out of harm's way: gangs, drugs, etc.

- Reverend Lamarr Goldman, youngest pastor of the ranks but is gung-ho and ready to go, establishing vital ministries: church redevelopment project, food pantry, youth ministry and community outreach groups

- Reverend Steve Daniels, Jr., a powerful pastor and celebrated as a man who has 'dedicated his life to preaching and teaching God's Word.' Sponsor of Immanuel Baptist Church in Monrovia, Liberia, sending medicine, food, tools, etc.

- Pastor Earl Nance, Jr., effective pastor who lends a spiritual and political hand in community work and outreach; multifaceted participant in several projects: National Baptist Convention, Board of Education, St. Louis Clergy Coalition and mediator with large companies for jobs for ex-offenders

- Reverend Isaac C. McCullough, effectual wearer of many hats: Chief Facilitator of "Breaking the Silence" and "Keeping it Real" workshops, aimed at creating dialogue on sex and sexuality issues in faith-based environments; member of The Black Church Initiative. Also works with St. Louis Health and Mental Health Depts.

- Reverend Andrew Latchison, Jr., a powerful 'preacher's preacher'; local, national and international ministry affiliations; creator of "BodyBuilders"®, a church- and people-empowering model; the 'original' nursing home and prison minister

I felt the need to list these great leaders in the order in which they responded. *Responding* is what they do. *Responding* is who they are. Vibrant meaning is added by them to Christ's directive: *"Go ye therefore, and teach all nations... Teaching them to observe all things whatsoever I have commanded you"* (Matthew 28:19,20).

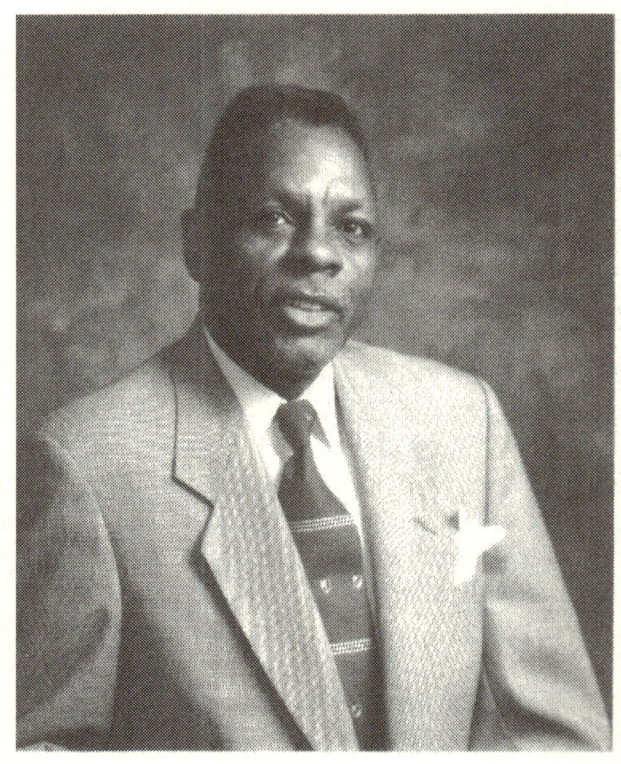

Reverend Charles M. Roach
Pastor of Trinity Mount Carmel Baptist Church
A.A., B.A., Masters in Education
27 years in Ministry, 16 years as Pastor
Married 34 years (Delores)

"A Pastor's Response to the AIDS Crisis"

Reverend Charles M. Roach

There is a crisis in communicable disease in our community, especially among the Black people. This crisis exists because there is a crisis in human behavior. No disease can become pandemic unless there be a certain human behavior that's promoting such an outcome.

Now the bible teaches that there is "nothing new under the sun" (Ecclesiastes). As we so well know, mankind has experienced various outbreaks of diseases, as long as we can remember. We have conquered many of these through medical breakthrough, treatment and medications. We have also benefited greatly through education and change of behaviors. We cannot expect to win any battle with disease unless there be a change in human behavior.

In our efforts to understand the dynamics of our fight to conquer the AIDS virus, we must emphasize the great need to change human behaviors. Since we know how a disease is spread and that it can be spread through *specific* human behaviors, then it follows that one would disengage mercy from that behavior, which would cause him to be a victim. Now, I know this seems to be so very basic but perhaps, just perhaps, this is indeed the answer to our problem.

As a cleric I am mandated not to teach or promote what is called "safe sex." The biblical guide is to teach and promote sex in the context of spiritual guidelines. The bible only approves of sex between male and female, and that this is to be done in the bonds of matrimony only. To do otherwise, according to biblical teachings, falls into the realm of sin. Sin in this case can be defined as the misappropriation of that which God has given. Sex between a man and woman in the bond of matrimony is good. It is good in its practice and good in the context that God has planned.

I realize that there are different ways one can be infected with the virus. However, if we just stopped and thought through the path of transmission, we would trace its beginning back to an inappropriate human behavior on somebody's part. This is my position on the problem.

Now allow me to offer a remedy to this problem. This is what I have come to believe to be true; others think differently. As a pastor having to deal with a gamut of human issues -- all having their negative impact on our community -- I've had to discover something that absolutely works. For me, in order to change behaviors that impact in harmful ways, one must adopt new behaviors. This is what the God of the bible offers every man and woman who will hear. The bible is not just a book of "don't do". On the contrary, it is a guide for experiencing a prosperous, healthy life. Its instructions are not given to make life a burden but to give us a *freedom* to do the things that will positively enhance every area of life.

One of my favorite instructions is found in Galatians 6:7: Be not deceived; God is not mocked: for whatsoever a man soweth, *that* shall he also reap. Now this principle works in the negative as well as the positive. What I mean is you can sow wrong behaviors and you can only expect to reap bad results. Thank God, you can sow right/good behaviors and you can expect right/good results. The choice is up to the individual. The other part of this instruction says, "And let us not be weary in well doing: for in due season we shall reap, if we faint not."

In conclusion, Galations 6:9 says to us don't grow tired of doing what's good and what's right according to God's standards. For when the time is right for you to have God's best, you will be in a position to receive His best -- but *take care* you don't give up on God's ways or on yourself to change wrong behaviors. He has promised His help!

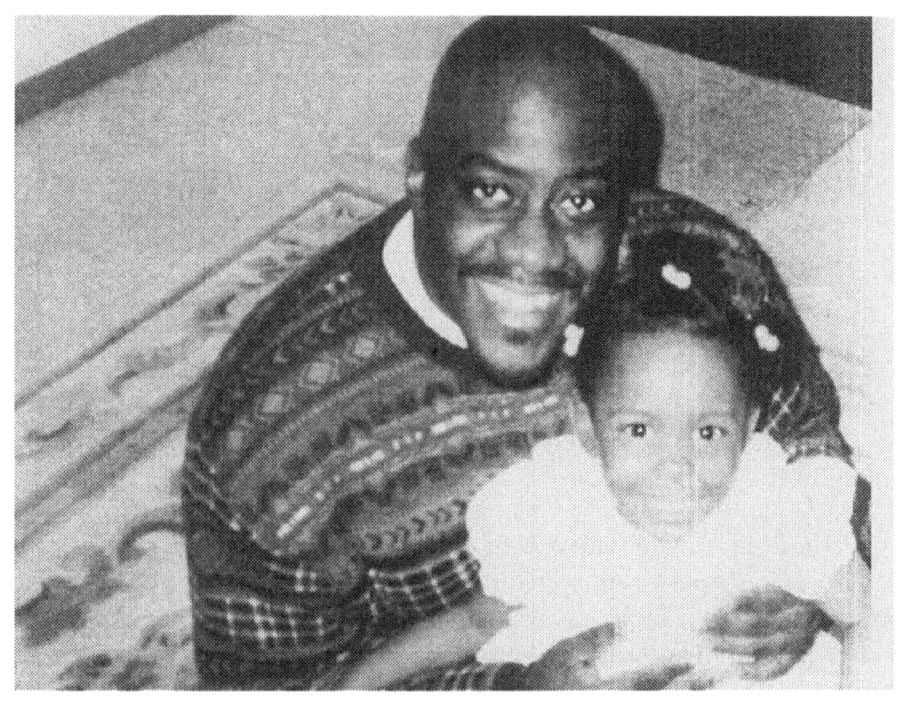

Minister Samson N. Latchison
(pictured here with 3 year old Esther Ruth)
In Ministry since the age of 14
Organizer of a "Coffee House" Ministry for college students; conducts
lectures. Works with troubled, violent and/or mentally challenged
youth. Partners with various outreach ministries; has ministered in
Cape Town, South Africa and Guatemala

"SOLUTIONS"...

Minister Samson N. Latchison

At the genesis of the Decade of Decadence (the 80's), came a nemesis to a sexually casual society that sang with Tina Turner *"What's Love Got To Do With It?"* I can recall hearing of Sunday School teachers, church musicians, athletes, and actors all falling prey to a disease which for many exposed their darkest secret and robbed them of their most precious gift -- life. The disease was AIDS.

I cannot empathize effectively with those who contracted this disease intravenously. I cannot empathize effectively with heterosexuals who contracted this disease from a dishonest partner. I can empathize with those viewed by many as the villainous carriers of this disease -- the gay community.

As a black male with a strong religious affiliation and a sexual orientation that opposes that affiliation, I have a unique perspective. The black community is being ravaged in pandemic proportions by AIDS. How dare we ask why! The cornerstone of the black community has always been the church. It is at the heartbeat of a people whose destiny in this country has always been less than secure. The black church is not immune to the devastation of AIDS. On the contrary, the church has lost many of her finest musicians, ministers, teachers, and laymen to this disease. Yet, the black church has worn a blindfold of pretension, her freshly-washed hands (though dripping with blood) are folded in a gesture of apathy and her feet stand firmly placed on doctrines and protocol.

I can easily recall having encounters of the gay culture -- not in bars or porno houses -- but in church. These often fervent, passionate, gifted people were those I saw most often in the choir stand and behind the "sacred desk". Due to the positions they held in various areas of the church, their sexuality was either ignored or just something everyone joked about but never dealt with appropriately. Suddenly, when the AIDS virus came with an indiscriminate, withered hand, first to the gay community (due to promiscuity) the only response to their swift demise was, "See, I told you they were gay!" No ministries were established, accountability became no more essential, education was not implemented and AIDS victims died alone and even when it was known these victims died of AIDS, their death was said to be caused by pneumonia.

When will the black church cease this immature game of "Hide and Seek"? When will we address the gay issue in our congregations with something more than "God created Adam and Eve, not Adam and Steve?" When will we provide AIDS education from a godly perspective instead of complaining about "safe sex" education? Has anyone realized that we have done less than any other nationality to deal with this disease and it remains one of the leading causes of death among Blacks?

What *is* the solution? Pastors, you must begin to develop ministries to the men of your congregations. Train your adult men to become better fathers and better husbands. Assist them in dealing with issues of physical and sexual abuse, which may have occurred from *their* fathers. Establish accountability groups, which foster honesty and loving confrontation. From these "fellowships of the heart" men can begin to experience intensive and extensive healing not limited to a Sunday morning worship service.

Gays are allowed to "come out of the closet" in every facet of society, except the church. Though we are usually well informed of those who are gay in our congregations, the "squeaky-clean" facade of religion makes hypocrites ("bad actors") of us all. Thus, gays are left unaccountable and while they are allowed to minister publicly, they remain sexually impure privately. When Jesus heals the leper in Mark chapter 1, He does the unthinkable by touching the leper's sores. Jesus spoke healing in many cases, but Jesus dares to touch "the untouchable". Can we do less and call ourselves His followers? Is the environment of the black church conducive to provide for the needs of struggling gays who are not "delivered"? Are there support groups in place for those bound in this sexual addiction? Or would we rather preach the annual "Instead of coming out of the closet, why don't you just clean it?!" sermon without extending a hand to touch them at the depth of their self-destructive behavior?

Is the black church ready to realize the delicate juxtaposition of our reality and God's truth? My reality is by sexual orientation I am tempted to be gay. God's truth declares that homosexuality is a sin. I am tempted to have sex with men. Though I attempt to resist that temptation, would I be chronically labeled "fag" and left to my own devices for spiritual survival in the black church? Yes, and worst yet, every "closet gay" in the church, though they testify of deliverance before the masses, would be at my doorstep for a "close encounter"! How do I know this to be true? Been there, done that! For far too long, the black church has redefined faith as denial. Paul in Romans chapter 7 clearly stated his reality: "I do not understand what I do. For what I want to do I do not do, but what I hate I do." Paul in Romans chapter 8, clearly stated God's truth: "No, in all these things we are more than conquerors through Him who loved us." Pastors, we must allow those struggling with homosexuality to say so as we allow "the redeemed of the Lord" to say so! Only then will there be hope for the former to fully realize the latter.

AIDS education must become part of our Sunday School curriculum. Historically, the church was the place where many pioneer children learned their ABC's. Abraham Lincoln's first reading textbook was The Bible. The parishioners of the black church deserve to know the "naked truth" about AIDS coupled with the Gospel truth from God. Four years ago, I taught AIDS education in Mannenberg, South Africa (a township of Cape Town) and Pastor Jerome Camphor of Jezreel Fellowship Church in Mannenberg said to me, "You as Americans would rather deal with the AIDS pandemic in Africa than deal with the AIDS pandemic in America." Today I realize we taught South African children in schools what Black children should have been taught in churches.

My dear brothers and sisters in Christ, until we are ready to be honest with this pandemic before God and before each other and lovingly deal with each other accordingly, prepare your best black suit or dress for numerous funerals to come -- or maybe your own...

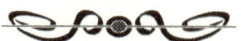

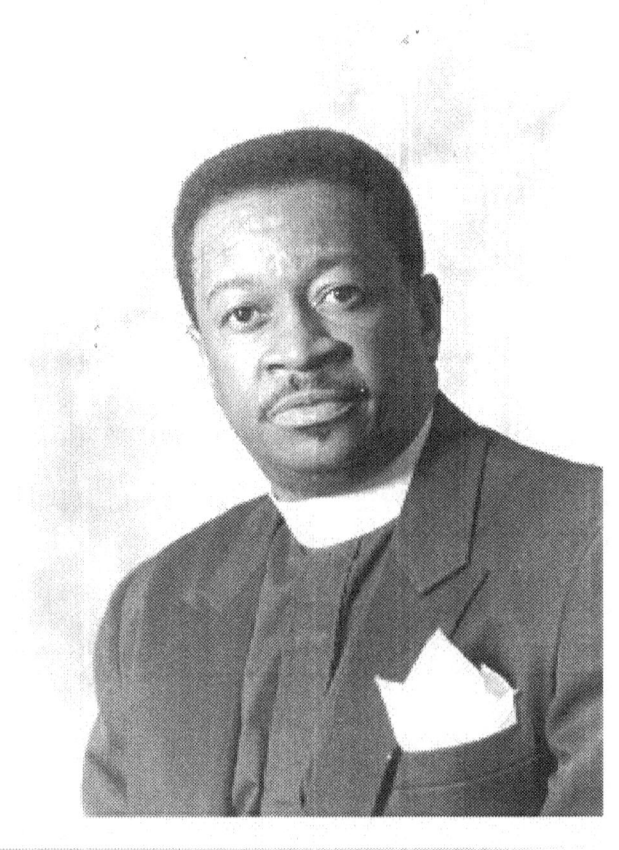

Archbishop Michael A. West, Sr.
Pastor of St. Michael's Temple of the Expanded Mind
Spiritual/Non-denominational
B.S., Masters in Theology, Ph.D., Ed. D.
Founder of St. Michael's Institute of Theology
Masons, Educational Assoc., Funeral Directors Assoc., Fraternities
51 years in Ministry, 37 years as Pastor
Married (Martha)

"Confusion, Conflict, Conquering"

Archbishop Michael A. West, Sr.

Regrettably, it has not yet dawned on "the Church" that "the Body of Christ" has AIDS. With the governance of our denominational and non-denominational bodies being headed by some of the most erudite and 'literally prepared' individuals, we yet are grappling with the **confusion** of what HIV/AIDS is all about!

The **confusion** of stigmatizing one group or another above and beyond another is still far too rampant in our supposed enlightened society and certainly in the Body of Christ, God's representative on Earth. Be not confused, HIV/AIDS is here now. Look at the multiplicity of our society and culture that has been affected in life, and certainly the large numbers claimed by death.

I listened at a funeral service of an 'otherwise' fine young man, to a minister whose apparent **confusion** led him to berate the homosexual lifestyle but throughout his discourse, failed to relate the hope, help or compassion that comes from Christ. It catapulted me into the thought process that made me examine his possible **confusion** that brought him to such **conflict**. **Conflict** -- not of what he was saying -- but **conflict** of soul, that as a 'man of God' he could not empathize and sympathize with the broader picture: this pandemic in our society and the chronic hurt of these and so many other people who must face certain events of its aftermath.

From years of study I've learned **confusion** is natural, **conflict** is always possible but until we can confront the real issue, there can be no real resolve (**conquering**)! The resolution of which I speak in terms of is **conquering** this 'demon spirit' called HIV/AIDS.

The Church has been in our society a main point of focus in educating, as well as, inspiring men and women. We have fallen asleep on 'our watch.' Our 'watch commander' will hold us accountable for not being alert and on task. We were told "Go ye therefore, and teach all nations, baptizing them in the name of the Father, and of the Son, and of the Holy Ghost: teaching them to observe all things whatsoever I have commanded you" (Matthew 28:19-20). We were told, "Neither do men light a candle and hide it under a bushel, but on a candlestick and it giveth light unto all in the house" (Matthew 5:15).

We were told by our Commander, "Occupy 'til I come!" HIV/AIDS can be **conquered** with the help of God through the forward move of the Church to educate thoroughly. It is not just the matter of the sacred sex method (abstinence until marriage) but recognizing that safe sex is *plausible* as well, through partnering with all of the key elements of society that truly believe it can be **conquered** -- and not be side-tracked by other prejudicial agendas that so often exist.

> "**IF** I shut up heaven that there be no rain, or
> **IF** I command the locusts to devour the land, or
> **IF** I send pestilence (disease, a.k.a., AIDS) among my people;
> **IF** my people which are called by my name, shall humble themselves, and
> pray, and seek my face, and turn from their wicked ways;
> **THEN** will I hear from heaven, and will forgive their sin, and will heal
> their land."
> **II Chronicles 7:13-14**

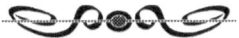

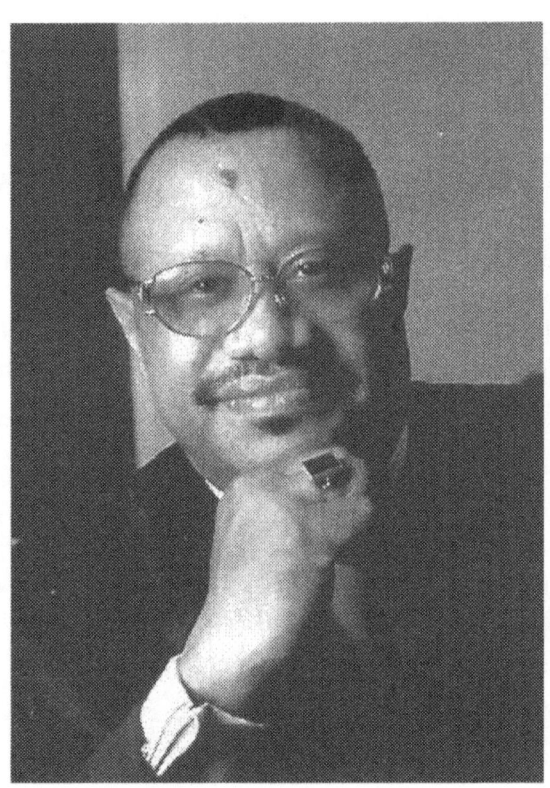

Bishop George White, Jr.
Pastor of West End Mount Carmel Full Gospel Baptist Church
Full Gospel/Baptist
**B. S., retired from St. Louis Police Dept.; detective and sergeant;
gubernatorial appointee to the Department of Mental Health Regional
Advisory Council Drug and Alcohol Abuse, as Chairman Emeritus of
Committed Caring Faith Communities (target cities faith organization of
Missouri), as Board of Directors of Faith House, as Vice President of the
Board of Directors of New Beginnings Treatment Center, and as a Board
Member of AACID Committee (African American Churches in Dialogue);
as Chairman of the Board for the West End Mount Carmel Community
Outreach Center, a board member for St. Louis for Kids, and is Advisory
Board Chairman for Ask Seek Knock Ministries, Inc.; 17 years as pastor;
Married (Sharon)**

The Results are in:
America is HIV/AIDS Positive...
and
<u>*Where*</u> In the World Is The Church?

Bishop George White, Jr.

There are well over 40 million people currently living with HIV/AIDS. HIV/AIDS is a global pandemic claiming 8,000 lives a day in some of the poorest and even the richest countries in the world. In 2003 alone there were:

- 5 million new infections. 700,000 of them were children under age 15
- 3 million AIDS-related deaths
- 2.5 million children living with HIV/AIDS, who are under age 15

HIV/AIDS is a plague of monumental proportions and is no longer confined to the original population o f men having sex with men. Children, women, heterosexuals, unborn babies, Christians, non-Christians, and people of every faith are getting hit hard by this disease and the numbers in the Black community are even more staggering.

It amazes me that I belong to a faith that proclaims that everything we need is set in the body of Christ, yet we are usually the last group of people to respond to world pandemics. I would venture to even say that 90% or more of the Pastors all over the world haven't a *clue* of the number of individuals right in their own churches that are suffering from this disease. Sermons about how to avoid AIDS are good but usually provide no comfort, compassion, or solution to those already infected with the virus. Have we ever really stopped to think that the 40 million individuals infected are *40 million souls* and the word of God clearly tells us that EVERY soul is precious in the sight of God. Shouldn't these souls also be precious in *our* sight?

As Christians, we haven't provided significant leadership in the fight against AIDS. We have been outraged and unified in our fight against the pandemic levels of black on black crimes, gang violence, the crack cocaine pandemic, and even the growing threat of terrorism with the recent September 11, 2002, terrorist attack. We must come to realize that the devil does not care how he destroys us and unless we use the same level of response and commitment to defeat AIDS as we do with every other weapon of warfare from the devil, we will all lose... As Christians, we have so much to contribute, yet our family, friends and community are dying at alarming numbers every day in the hands of the enemy, right before our very eyes.

The Call

I believe that there is no better place for HIV/AIDS victims to heal than the church. We have the influence, the authority, and the capacity to reach these individuals in a community of faith, hope, love and even miracles. Since the church is usually one of the first places that most people turn for help in times of trouble, it is imperative that we become better prepared. However, we must become willing to shift our seats from judgment to service. Now I must interject, that yes, we have come a long way in the faith community. Often, without prejudice, we serve the homeless, the crack addict, and the prostitute and have mastered the art of providing the love, hope and forgiveness needed to help these folks heal. We are no stranger to people who may or may not have sinned, yet are ill from a disease or simply from the result of poor choices. The numbers are too high for us to continue to gamble, theorize, blame or remain fear-stricken or dumb-founded in this arena. We must rise from the shock that this disease is killing – not only the community – but our own church members as well, and adopt the serenity prayer to gain the strength to be at the forefront of this battle. The serenity prayer simply says:

"God grant us the serenity to accept the things I cannot change, courage to change the things I can – and the wisdom to know the difference."

We can begin with some simple dialogue. The topics that I believe we are all equipped to handle in the faith community include: caring for the sick, the dying, the orphans of AIDS-related death victims, prevention training and education and spiritual counseling.

"People who are living with HIV constitute a minority. Society has responded to their plight with intense prejudice. They have been subject to systemic disadvantage and discrimination. They have been stigmatized and marginalized. Society's response has forced many of them not to reveal their HIV status for fear of prejudice. This in turn has deprived many of them of the help they would otherwise have received. People living with HIV or AIDS are one of the most vulnerable groups in our society." The Constitutional Court – Hoffman vs. South African Airways

The church must stop responding like the secular world. Our focus must not be on whether this is the wrath of God or a reaping of sinful choices for people involved in negative behaviors. We should instead be asking why has God sent or allowed such a challenge to serve masses of dying people under our watch. We must rise to the challenge and ask ourselves, "What would Jesus do?" I've never read in all my studies where Jesus passed by a group of sick people without so much as offering to serve them. Not knowing what to do can no longer be used as an excuse. Sometimes Jesus just asked people, "What would you have me to do?" This simple phrase may be all that is needed to begin a foundation of health, hope, and healing for these souls. We *can* make a difference!

The Challenge

The stigma and discrimination against HIV/AIDS victims are two of the major obstacles to effective HIV/AIDS prevention and care. Fear of discrimination may prevent people from acknowledging their HIV/AIDS status publicly. People with HIV/AIDS may have already been turned away from health care services, denied housing and employment, shunned by their friends and colleagues, and turned down for insurance coverage. In some cases, they may be evicted from home by their families, divorced by their spouses, rejected by their children, and some may have even suffered physical violence. The church has become their last hope. If we are not willing to change our walk and our talk in this matter, the stigma attached to HIV/AIDS may extend into the next generation, placing an emotional burden on innocent children who may also be trying to cope with the death of a parent from this disease.

Only by confronting stigma and discrimination will the fight against HIV/AIDS be won. The challenge facing us as Christians is to support people who are infected and affected by HIV/AIDS. As Christians and as Church leaders we have a duty to be aggressive learners in this arena and explicit teachers about the nature and causes of this disease. We need to help break the stigma and the silence surrounding this disease and thus enable people living with HIV/AIDS to have adequate and essential support. We must begin to dispel the many myths that surround HIV/AIDS-infected individuals. One of the most incorrect myths is that people suffering from HIV/AIDS are silent because of shame. The truth is that communities and the church have silenced these individuals by not being a compassionate environment where people are free to tell their stories. This myth tells us a lot about our own prejudices and lack of compassion for people where it is simply accepted that some people must stay outside the possibility of receiving healing, in silent anguish. The mere fact that the church can remain in denial without embracing people locked away in the dark trenches of silent suffering, points to the acceptance of prejudice and injustice against certain things. This attitude, if left unchecked, will lead us right to the death of our reputation, power, and effectiveness toward a world of people who need us the most.

The Truth

We all have skeletons in our closet, stories to tell, and a history that brought many of us running through the church doors, beaten and bruised from the consequences of our past. These stories, testimonies and phenomenal healings are the exact reason that Jesus came to show us how to embrace all people of our community. Without these stories there would be no need of the "Great Physician" which is our Lord and Savior, Jesus Christ. From these stories the wisdom of life is passed on from one generation to the next. But silencing people says that some stories are unimportant to God, feared by the church, and therefore, not allowed to be told. Silencing some stories has a negative effect – not just on the church – but on the community because through silence, lies and deception continue to destroy our lives. This is the fertile soil for all forms of sin and prejudice to thrive. When the story of HIV/AIDS does not become part of the story of a community and church, when we do not allow it to become "our story", we ourselves are not free, but remain hypocritical, broken and in bondage. Silence is the theology of death and destruction and embraces hypocrisy on the deepest level. But the Bible tells a different story -- a story of hope, health, healing and justice for all who are suffering and in need of a transformed life.

"Through our silence, many churches share responsibility for the fear that has swept our world more quickly than the virus itself. Sometimes churches have hampered the spread of accurate information, or created barriers to open discussion and understanding. Sometimes they have reinforced racist attitudes by neglecting issued of HIV/AIDS because it occurs predominately among certain ethnic or racial groups, who may be unjustly stigmatized as the most likely carriers of the infection." – A WCC Study Document, pg. 5.

"The situation calls for a fresh resolve by churches to address the challenge of HIV/AIDS directly… It is the churches themselves which are affected by HIV/AIDS, and their credibility depends on the way in which they respond. They are confronted with people, members of the body of Christ, who not only seek support and solidarity, but who ask: Do you want to be my brother and sister?" Ibid

I challenge every reader today to take a real hard look at these facts and ask yourself, how long do you think it will take for us to be completely destroyed by our own unwillingness to change?

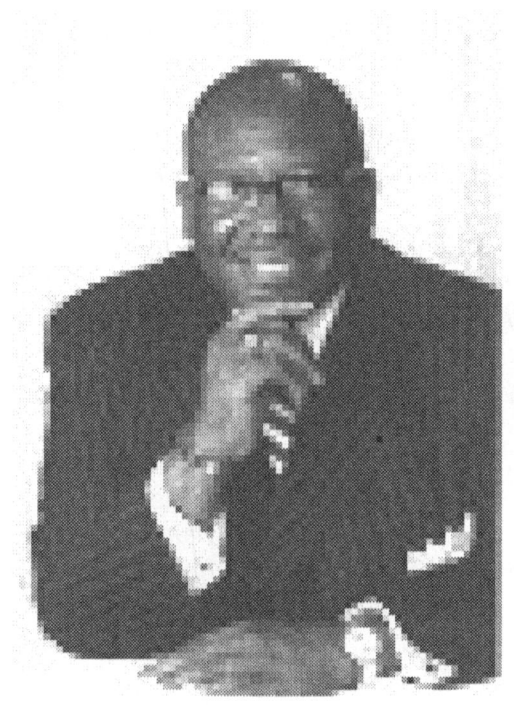

Bishop Dr. Wyatt I. Greenlee, Jr.

Pastor of The Greater New Higher Heights Christian Church
United Church of Christ
B.S. (Business Administration), Masters (Education Administration),
Ph.D. (Education Administration); Pastoring 25 years
Affiliations: Fellowship 2000, T.D. Jakes (Aaron's Army), Global
Missions Board, UCC, W.S.P.D., Exhortation-Presiding Bishop/Prelate

W.W.J.D   or   W.<u>D</u>.J.D
What Would Jesus Do?   What <u>*Did*</u> Jesus Do?

Bishop Wyatt I. Greenlee

The Catholics initiated a great campaign. It was called W.W.J.D. (What Would Jesus Do?) But in light of the HIV/ AIDS pandemic, I hear another campaign called W.D.J.D. (What <u>Did</u> Jesus Do?) I do believe some people would be literally shocked concerning Jesus' response to this disease.

After ministering in South Africa and the U.S.A, I have noted that four major barriers hinder ministry in the midst of the AIDS pandemic fear: its perception as a "sinner's disease," its link to human sexuality and its terminal nature. As Christians, however, we are called to overcome these barriers, for the sake of persons in need. For this to happen, we must sense a strong central motivation for such a ministry. There is one compelling motivation for certain in the midst of the AIDS crisis: Compassion. Our ministerial response to this disease crisis is part, as we are gripped by Godly compassion.

Compassion is crucial for genuine ministry, although this emotion is not readily present, nor easily developed in contemporary society. In fact, total compassion is beyond the ability of humans to produce. True compassion is a divine trait and is present in the world only as the fruit of the Holy Spirit is manifest in the lives of believers. If compassion is to be present, we must open ourselves to the working of the Holy Spirit. A first stop toward the fulfillment of this challenge is taken when we come to understand more fully the divine compassion we are called to emulate.

The obvious beginning place lies in the meaning of the concept itself. Compassion means literally "to suffer with." This forms the background to a standard dictionary definition: "a sympathetic emotion created by the misfortunes of another, accompanied by a desire to help."

Compassion for others in the face of their misfortunes does not arise in a vacuum, however. Its source lives in a more foundational emotion or truth -- love that is *agape* -- whereby persons give of themselves unconditionally for the sake of others. Such love is seldom experienced in our world -- not even in the church. On the contrary, a perfect example of this emotion and truth can be found always in the compassionate love shown to us by God. This love is not performance based. Neither does it have respect of person. It is for this reason Christians look to divine revelation of God in Jesus Christ. There they discover the loving, compassionate nature of God. As we come to view the perfect love of God, the Holy Spirit is able to create in us the kind of compassionate love needed for ministry in the midst of crisis, such as the AIDS pandemic.

A persistent theme in the Bible is the presentation of God as the 'Compassionate One', according to Christian theology. Love is the foundational moral attribute of God. Love is visible in a primary way with the Godhead, for God is the Triune One -- the community of Father, Son and Holy Spirit. These three Trinitarian persons constitute One God, in that they are bound together by the cord of divine love.

John, the Apostle of Love, characterizes God in this way. In his first epistle, John makes a simple, yet profound declaration. "God is love . . ." (1 John 4:16) Love which describes God's own essence, also characterizes God's relationship to creation. Because God is love, God loves the world. Again John describes this love for us: "For God so loved the world that He gave His one and only Son . . ." (John 3:16). God relates to the world out of the Abundance of His own character, which is Love.

This formulation -- God as abounding in love and filled with compassion -- is found repeatedly throughout the Old Testament, forming as it were a central faith affirmation concerning the divine nature (Nehemiah 9:7, Psalms 86:15, 103:8, 111:4, 116:5, 145:8, Isaiah 54:10, Joel 2:13). Because of the divine love, the plight of all God's creatures evokes compassion from God. Not only does the Old Testament declare God to be the Compassionate One; it also links this compassion to the human predicament. This ideal is bound up with the Hebrew word that speaks of compassion: Racham. This term expresses a deep and tender feeling as is aroused by the sight of weakness or suffering in those that are dear to us or need our help. Racham, or "compassion" also portrays the response that arises when the divine love views the struggles of God's people.

Divine compassion leads to divine action. According to the New Testament, however, the supreme action that rose out of the divine compassion is the salvation available in Jesus Christ. That this event is the expression of God's mercy is reiterated throughout its pages. A specially beautiful declaration of this truth is found in the book of Ephesians: "But because of this great love for us, God, who is rich in mercy, made us alive with Christ even when we were dead in transgressions -- it is by grace you have been saved." (Ephesians 2:4-5)

Jesus' compassion expressed itself in ministry. As He saw the needs of people around Him -- needs that sparked His emotions -- Jesus did not stand aside. On the contrary, He engaged in action to alleviate the misery of the people and minister to their needs. To those who had been sick, Jesus healed their diseases. (Matthew 4:23, 9:35, 14:14, 19:2) In His memory, Jesus was not afraid to make physical contact with those in need. He was not afraid to touch the outcast of His day, those suffering from the dreaded and contagious disease of leprosy. (Matthew 8:3). This debilitating illness exacted an impenetrable wall between the afflicted and the society of the healthy, much like AIDS does today. Laws against any kind of contact with lepers were strictly enforced and the victims of this disease were treated as the living dead. One man, however, was willing to cross the barriers and touch these outcasts -- Jesus. The willingness of the Master to touch those to whom he ministered becomes more significant when it is remembered that actual physical contact was not necessary for Jesus to heal. He had the power to cure the sick without the least amount of physical contact or even physical presence. (Luke 7:1-10) Nevertheless, He freely chose to touch the untouchable. These acts demonstrate Jesus' great compassion.

According to the Bible, the compassionate nature of God is revealed in God's actions in history, climaxing in the coming of Jesus Christ. This central attribute of the divine nature places a great responsibility on Christ's church. As God's people, we are to be emulators of the compassionate love. His example calls us to be the compassionate one and to reflect the divine character.

W.D.J.D - What Did Jesus Do? He showed compassion to us all. As Christians, we are compelled by the divine compassion to minister to those in need, including persons struggling with AIDS. Our task must, therefore, begin with prayerful and conscious attempts to be sensitive to the presence, working, and filling of the Holy Spirit in our lives and in our churches.

We must rise to the challenge and be who we are called to be: the loving compassionate people of God, who serve others to the glory of God and for the sake of suffering people.

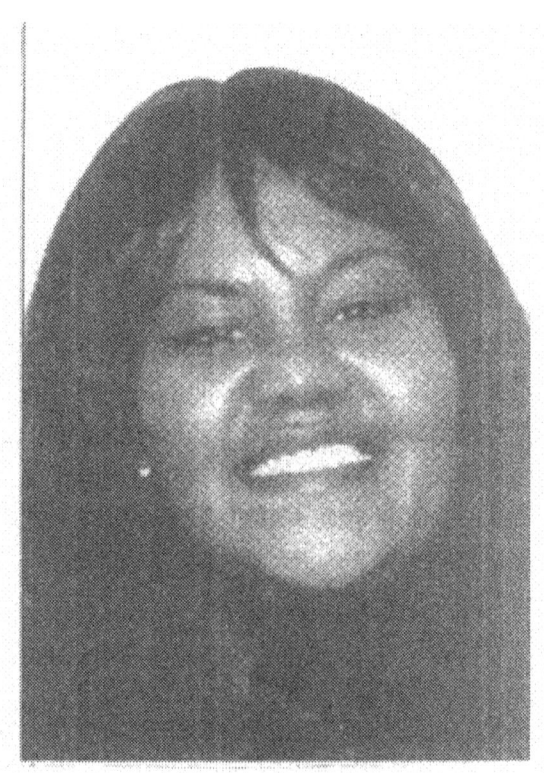

Evangelist Ruth Latchison Nichols
Youth on the Move Crusade, Inc.
Gospel Singer 42 years, Stage Performer ("Be Careful What You Pray
For"), "Isle of Dreams" (formerly "The Revelation")
Spiritual Counselor; Nursing Home and Senior Ministry; Prison
Ministry; Youth Ministry for 14 years;
in Evangelistic Ministry 24 years
Married (Rev. Sam Nichols)

"LEAVE THE CHILDREN ALONE!"

Evangelist Ruth Latchison Nichols

The Bible states in II Chronicles 7:13c, 14: "...*or if I send a pestilence among the people;*

If my people which are called by my name shall humble themselves, and pray and seek my face, and turn from their wicked ways then will I hear from heaven and will forgive their sin and heal their land." It is important to read more than one verse of a chapter to get a complete understanding of what is being inferred. According to Webster's dictionary 'pestilence' is defined as a 'deadly or virulent disease; something regarded as harmful or destructive.' In other words: AIDS...

I must say that as we point fingers at the homosexual, the intravenous drug user, etc. to say 'it is their fault' and they are 'getting what they deserve', what do we do about the faithful wife or husband who acquires the disease due to the infidelity of a spouse – not necessarily with a homosexual encounter but with *heterosexual* encounters? The result can be totally catastrophic to eventually millions. According to statistics this is exactly the scenario being played out, which has caused this disease to reach the pandemic. No one is immune to it. *No one...* So let us look realistically and truthfully at our position. It is time that we take a look – not on the *outside* – but *within* the church.

As ministers and ambassadors of the Word of God, we must preach repentance, confession of sins and acceptance of Jesus Christ as Savior. Yes, it is correct that God is able to deliver and set free, to make all things new, to reconcile and restore us to Himself. However, it is also equally necessary that in being effective in last-day ministry that we become transparent, accountable and responsible for our actions and be *real* about where we are. The 'church" is as it was during the time of Jesus, with Pharisees and Sadducees still prevalent. We are still judgmental and self-righteous, but yet participating and even *orchestrating* many of the inappropriate sexual behaviors that have brought us to this pandemic place!

Suppose, just suppose (go with me, I'm going somewhere with this...) that the woman who was caught in the act of adultery and about to be stoned according to Jewish law, being brought to Jesus who immediately made the famous statement: "Let he who is without sin cast the first stone". We know that the people dropped their stones and walked away. But what if one of Jesus' disciples had said to her: "He spared you from death, now you *owe* him. Meet him in one hour at the local inn and there you can *show* him how much you appreciate what he did for you." Suppose that had happened? That woman would have not been able to walk with Jesus as she walked in her deliverance and towards wholeness to become one of the greatest testimonies of all times.

Sadly, that is the situation in many of our religious institutions. I have now been walking in my deliverance from intravenous drug use for 23 years. But 23 years ago, I contacted some prominent leaders of churches ('friends' of the family) and requested money to try and get the 'monkey off my back.' Instead of ministering to me or denying me the money, they took advantage of the opportunity for a sexual encounter to say, "I scratched your back, now you scratch mine." They would give me what I wanted if I gave them what *they* wanted. Had I been infected with AIDS and had not had a fear of God as it relates to messing around within the church, not only would they have violated their homes but also would have been infected and as a result, infect their wives.

Let us realistically approach a solution to the problem. And if you're not part of the solution, you are part of the problem. Let us do away with the pompous, arrogant, self-righteous, judgmental behaviors which have perpetuated this disaster and move towards true deliverance: LEAVE THE CHILDREN ALONE!!! Molestation, sexual abuse, incest, rape (statutory or otherwise), child pornography -- *leave them alone...*

Much of the promiscuity of our youth does not start among themselves. Many times children are introduced to sex inappropriately by adults. Pornography, books, touching them in inappropriate places, taking advantage of a curious teenager (male or female) and exposing them to activities they have no business knowing about. This type of activity did not just begin. In my day, men were leading young girls to their demise but it was 'hush-hush' and children were not allowed to talk about adults.

Things wouldn't be quite as twisted as they are now because "hurt people, *hurt* people.'

Even in school I can remember teachers, counselors and administrators of every walk, 'hitting' on a teenage girl. How does a child tell its mother that the people she trusts to teach, nurture and protect her child are the perpetrators, are the criminal, sick, perverted, sadistic creatures – the virtual *monsters* in the closet or under the bed that every child fears when the lights go out? If every child came forth to demand justice (yesterday and now), there would be *no room* to house the perpetrators in the prison system – and it would *not* be just the Catholic priests.

Well, at 15 I was brutally gang-raped – a virgin, having dreamt of walking down the isle in a beautiful white dress… I was dragged into a filthy vacant house, thrown upon a filthy mattress and knocked unconscious. Several of my teeth were knocked out and my uterus was turned inside out by the violence. I left that place with a violent hatred I cannot explain, but which put me on a path of committing violence against others as a drug-addicted gang leader. This anger wreaked havoc on my life and upon anyone foolish enough to involve themselves with me. But thanks be to God for a praying mother and the grace of God!

II Chronicles 7:14 says, 'If my people which are called by my name (Christians, saints, etc.) would humble themselves (become transparent, share your testimony of deliverance or your walk towards deliverance). If you're yet dealing with some 'issues' let it be known. Truthfully, God is working on *all* of us; we all have some 'issues.' We always talk about the homosexual lifestyle but in Romans 1, verses 29 through 31, there are 22 *other* sins that will damn the soul, things we consider small: *"envy, murder, deceit, malice, whisperers, backbiters, proud, etc. They which commit such things are worthy of death."* We've got a long way to go to be like the Lord and cannot afford to point a finger at *anyone.* "Yea, *all* of you be subject one to another and be clothed with humility; for God resists the proud and gives grace to the humble" (I Peter 5:5).

It is time to remove the mask and just come *real.* Seek God's face and be truthful about where you are. Though men look on the outward appearance, God looks at the heart. True repentance is being sorry for our sins. Change what you can and those things you can stop doing, stop. Stay away from people who would tempt you and any environment that promotes evil. Draw close to God and He will draw close to you. Develop a true relationship based upon honesty and humility. God said, *"Then* will I *hear* from heaven, *I will forgive* their sin and *I will heal* the land"…

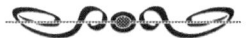

"Healing, The Will of God"

Dr. Ralph Petty, Sr.
Pastor of City of Refuge Christian Church

Jesus has already declared, "He has come to do His Father's will." It is the will of God that we the believers in Christ Jesus be healed and made whole by the work that was accomplished at Calvary. In 3 John 2 it is recorded, "Beloved, I wish above all things that thou may prosper and be in health, even as thy soul prospereth." When we begin to look at healing, we must find the will of God for the situation. The word 'will' is defined as a wish or desire often combined with determination; something desired, a choice or determination of one having authority or power.

Consider the word **'will'** in making the determination of healing. We can now see that it is the **'will'** (desire, choice or determination) of God that we are healed because of the price that has been paid by His son, Jesus the Christ.

Since Jesus came to do the Father's will and the Father's will is that we all be in health, healing is a promise to every believer. God's wish and desire -- coupled with determination -- is the ministry that Jesus Christ had on earth. Matthew 4:23 reads, "Jesus went throughout Galilee, teaching in their synagogues, preaching the good news of the kingdom, and healing every disease and sickness among the people." There was never a sickness or disease that Jesus felt that could not be healed. He knows the will of God for the people of God, and with a personal determination, He sat out to do the Father's will.

With knowing the will of the Father, the Son received **authority** and **power** to carry out the **will.** When someone has left you in charge of carrying out his or her will, you then have authority and power to do what you think is best for the estate. We as believers must do more than just know the will of God. We must take the will and <u>embrace it</u> with a determination to carry out the will that we have been appointed executors of. After receiving Jesus Christ into our lives we have then been given authority, and then, after receiving the Holy Spirit to dwell inside of us, we now have power to heal the sick. Matthew 10:1 reads, "He called his twelve disciples to Him and gave them authority to drive out evil spirits and to heal every disease and sickness." So as disciples today we have the same authority to heal the sick. I believe when what we know hooks up with a determination, we will begin to see a great move of healing in the land.

I pray that someday what we say from our mouths will really be in our hearts. Do we really believe that there is <u>nothing</u> too hard for God? The bible teaches us that Jesus went about healing <u>all</u> manner of sickness and disease. I believe that even in the outbreak of HIV and AIDS, there is still nothing too hard for God. There has been such a great stigma attached to this disease that not many have wanted to deal with it or be associated with it. Many have declared it to be a curse from God and, thus, we do nothing about it. God has never had a problem of getting rid of whatever or whomever He chose to get rid of. This disease has infected and affected our nation.

It is high time for us to be like Jesus -- to go about healing all manner of disease. It is the will of God that all people are in health -- not just those whom we deem to be worthy -- but to minister healing to all who are challenged in their health. We have the will.   So now let's execute it. HIV and AIDS is just like any other disease: it has to *bow* to the all-powerful name of Jesus Christ. Jesus healed all manner of sickness and I believe that HIV and AIDS is a part of that list, too. It is recorded in Malachi 4:2, "But for you who revere my name, the Son of Righteousness will rise with healing in its wings. And you will go out and leap like calves released from the stall."

The name of the Lord and the righteousness of the Lord is enough to release those who are challenged with this sickness. What a great testimony to God when our determination has caught up with our talk and people begin to be healed of this disease -- in the name of **Jesus!**

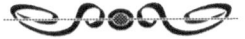

"The Church Must Stand for Righteousness"

Reverend Carl S. Smith, Sr.
Pastor of New Beginning Missionary Baptist Church
Married (Geraldine)

In the year 1619, blacks were brought to America on slave ships. We were abused and exploited by the oppressive society in which we were enslaved. The power of free choice was stripped from our ancestors and their bodies were used for sexual experiences in which they had no control. Our men were used as brute beast to create more slaves and our women were used as breeders, raped mercilessly by brutal slave owners.

As a result, silence about sexual issues within black families, black churches and black communities are the norm. Because of our negative experiences, sex is a taboo subject that belies our existence. Since sex has not been openly discussed, generations of black children have been raised with a 'slave mentality', believing that black males can seed woman after woman without responsibility or reprisal. Young black women desiring companionship feel that the greatest influence is their body, rather than a strong mind.

The Church has a responsibility to God and our young people to properly and morally educate. People perish for a lack of knowledge. With HIV and AIDS at pandemic levels, we must insist on moral abstinence from sex until marriage – and even then, marry only after the necessary testing has been performed.

The Church *must* stand for righteousness…

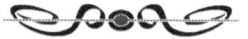

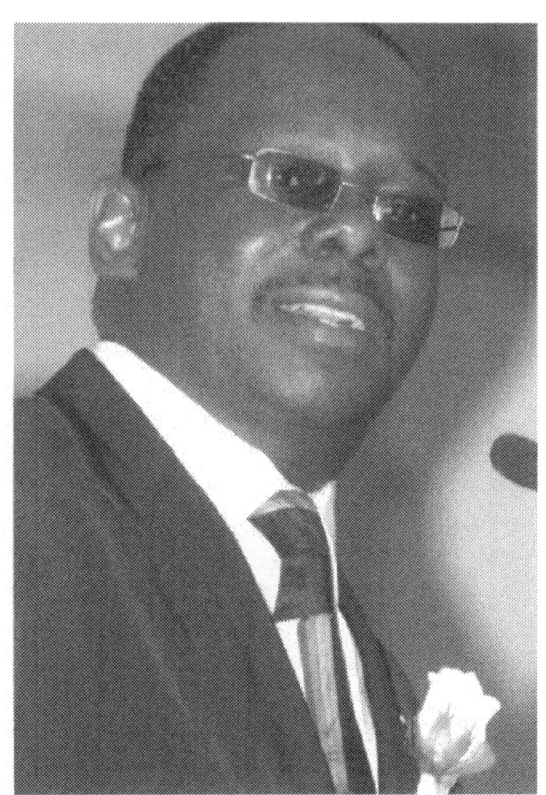

Reverend Lamarr Goldman

Pastor of Christ's Southern Mission Baptist Church
In Ministry 15 years; pastoring for 4 years
Member of certain Professional Organizations
Married (Beverly)

"Show Yourself to the Priest"

Reverend Lamarr Goldman

I would have to admit, I am a little uneducated in the matter of HIV/AIDS. The church is in need of education on the matter. However, I am sure that like any other disease that we may contract there *has* to be a cure for AIDS.

Being a preacher of the gospel, I must look at situations from the Word of God and not draw from my own conclusion on the matter. I believe in God's word, and that "there is *nothing* impossible with Him."

I draw from a story in the book of Luke 17:11-19: *"And it came to pass, as he went to Jerusalem that he passed through the midst of Samaria and Galilee. And as he entered into a certain village, there met him ten men that were lepers, which stood afar off. And they lifted up their voices and said, 'Jesus, Master, have mercy on us.' And when he saw them, he said to them: 'Go, show yourselves to the priests.' And it came to pass, that as they went, they were cleansed. And one of them when he saw that he was healed turned back, and with a loud voice glorified God. And fell down on his face at Jesus' feet, giving him thanks: and he was a Samaritan. And Jesus answered saying, 'Were there not ten cleansed? Where are the other nine? There is not found where they returned to give glory to God, except this one stranger. And he said unto him, 'Arise, go your. Your faith has made you whole."*

In biblical times, leprosy was a fatal disease that required a person to be put outside of the city. Individuals did not want to catch the disease and stayed away. We do the same thing to those that have HIV/AIDS, we put them at a distance. When the Lord focused on the ten, he related something to them that we need to project to those that have this deadly disease: *"Go, show yourselves to the Preacher."*

Why would Jesus, who healed all manner of sickness, tell the lepers to do such a thing? Could it be that in order for them to get back into the community, into society, they needed the blessing of the Priest of the town? Through obedience they were healed on their way.

Sometimes we are afraid of what others will say and will hide the problem from those that love us the most. Love will cover a multitude of sins. However, there is now such a problem with our society at large – wearing masks for so long that we are ashamed to take them off – afraid to risk the cruel opinions of others and the damage it causes our esteem.

But God can heal *all* manner of sickness and disease. All God requires is that we make a complete turn from the thing that has entrapped us. I would not allow the dirt from my past hinder *the healing* in my future.

We as a church must be careful of how we treat those with this disease. Whether the disease was contracted through immorality, birth or blood transfusion, it is a real problem that has plagued our society as a whole. It affects us *all*. However, we must turn to the Lord, get back to God -- who is the salvation of us all…

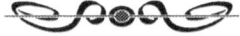

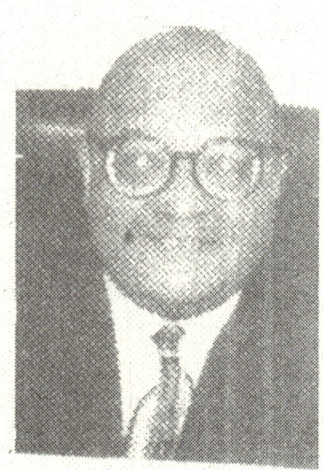

Reverend Earl E. Nance, Jr.

Greater Mount Carmel Missionary Baptist Church
Current pastor; served 15 years as Co-pastor under his father,
Civil rights activist Rev. Earl E. Nance, Sr., who pastored 43 years;
Member of St. Louis Board of Education (1987-1997);
Past President of the Missouri Progressive Baptist Convention;
Past President of the Progressive National Baptist Convention Midwest
Region Congress of Christian Education, serving as Dean;
Established four (4) schools in four year term
Currently serves on the following boards:
United Way of Greater St. Louis, St. Louis Science Center,
Mathews-Dickey Boys Club, Monsanto YMCA, St. Louis Sport
Commission of Metropolitan St. Louis; Former Education Liaison for
Mayor Francis Slay; Past President of St. Louis Clergy Coalition
(Married,Viola)

"The Effect of HIV/AIDS and Our Response"

Reverend Earl E. Nance, Jr.
Pastor of Mount Carmel Missionary Baptist Church

There is no question, or no argument alive that can challenge the fact of the devastation of AIDS in our world and in our community. It took a while for people to get over the stigma associated with AIDS during those early years. But thanks to Hall of Fame basketball player and businessman, Magic Johnson, we can freely talk and inform. Now, what can we do?

- (1) We can inform our church members about the real facts of HIV/AIDS

- (2) We can create a 'comfort zone' for people to talk openly about family members who may be affected

- (3) We can assign a liaison to work with effective programs to educate and reduce the risks

- (4) We can develop an action plan for our church or organization to act upon

We *CAN*...

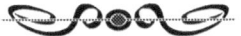

"No Blaming, No Judging. Know Only Love"

Ms. Sheila R. Grisby, BSN, MPH, RN
HIV/AIDS Program Coordinator ~ St. Louis

A small grass roots effort that began in St. Louis over nine years ago, has evolved to allow churches of all faith traditions to join together in working to bring about awareness and compassion to persons infected with and families affected by HIV/AIDS.

The "Black Church Week of Prayer for the Healing of AIDS" is a week-long celebration where churches of all denominations gather to highlight and focus on the role the Black Church can and should play in addressing HIV/AIDS within their faith walls. It is through awareness, education and compassion that we empower persons and families living with HIV and/or AIDS to be affirmed by their faith and be bold in their conviction that they, too, are worthy of all of God's blessings.

It is with this work that we have come to realize that we are called to a level of ministry that requires people who are open enough to know that all we are required to do as God's people is to love one another as He has loved us – a principle that sounds very simple but is our hardest commandment to keep. It is while we are trying to achieve this principle that we often find ourselves falling short because we get caught up in inflicting blame, judging others and their circumstance, or condemning others' lifestyles and choices.

We, as a Black community, have always depended heavily upon our faith and in the healing power of prayer. We know that prayer changes things. What we often fail to recognize, however, is that through sincere *prayer* and *patience* it also changes people. We have witnessed in the St. Louis metropolitan area the fruits of our labor. We have been consistent with our message and our pursuit of providing the tools for churches to address this issue within their own faith communities. We have seen the doors of churches open to address this issue because the needs are steadily increasing for persons and families being faced with this pandemic here in this area.

This disease now has a face. It is the face of our Black Family. The numbers are sobering, demonstrating to us that every aspect of our community is being impacted in some way. When we look at the cases within the metropolitan St. Louis area we find that Black men represented 41% of the total cases reported in 2003. While Black women represented 17% of the total reported cases of HIV, they represented 75% of the total number of women being reported with HIV in metropolitan St. Louis. The issue becomes even more astounding when we realize that persons who are 50 and older represent over 38% of the cases being seen here.

We encourage you to join in the fight to address this pandemic that has attacked our community and unite with us in being the catalyst to mobilize communities to respond compassionately to persons and families impacted by HIV/AIDS.

No blaming, no judging. Know only LOVE...

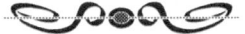

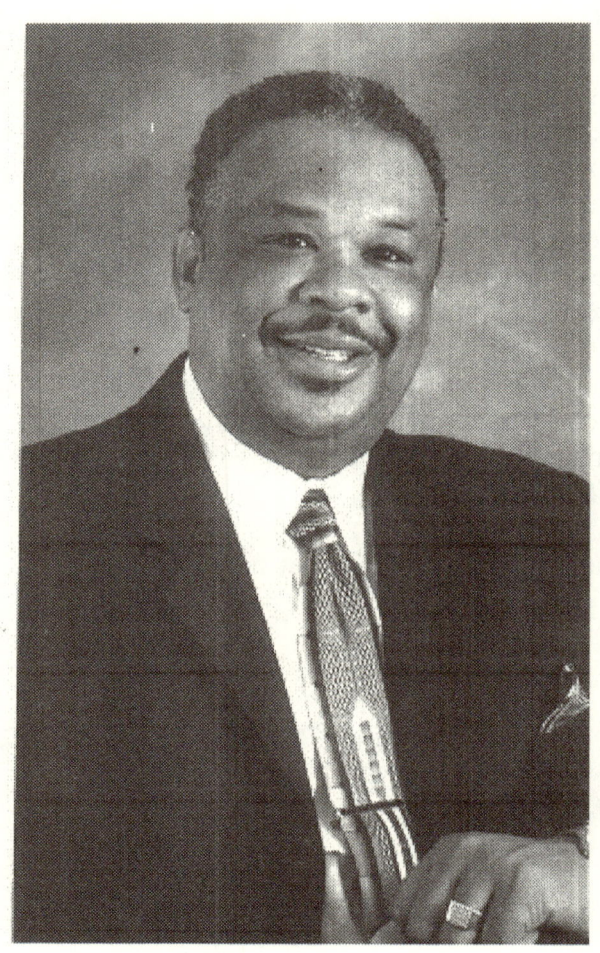

Reverend Steve Daniels, Jr.
Pastor of Shiloh Missionary Baptist Church ~ Minnesota
**B.A. Religious Education, Honorary Doctorate
In 1997 led National Baptist Convention, USA Inc. sponsored trip to
Holy Land and preached in Jerusalem; sponsors Immanuel Baptist
Church in Monrovia, Liberia; Who's Who in American Professionals
1996; NAACP
Married (Rosa) 33 years**

"There Is A Need"...

Reverend Steve Daniels, Jr.

Though blessed by God to have my ministry extend beyond American soil – Jerusalem, Monrovia, Liberia and other countries – *everywhere,* I have seen a need... This need extends far beyond the mere boundaries of ethnicity, denominational affiliation, education and economic standing. The need exist *everywhere* for self-control and self-examination, especially in light of the AIDS epidemic.

God's word declares in Ecclesiastes 3:1-7, "To *everything* there is a season and a time to every purpose under the heaven. There is a time to speak and a time to keep silent." For the church the time to speak is *now*. For the church the time for silence is *over*. For, while we were silent, someone became a victim of domestic violence. While we were silent, a young woman or young man became a victim of sexual abuse. While we were silent, teens explored their sexuality in seedy squalor. Somewhere, someone became infected with AIDS. While we were silent, questions needed to be asked and answered. But because no one was around to lend an ear or a hand, another young person surrendered to peer pressure.

As faith leaders, we are mandated to lead by example, by prayer, by counsel and by the Word of God. Let us be committed in fulfilling the Great Commission on earth, and in doing whatever it takes to engage all humankind in right-thinking and life enhancing choices...

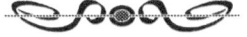

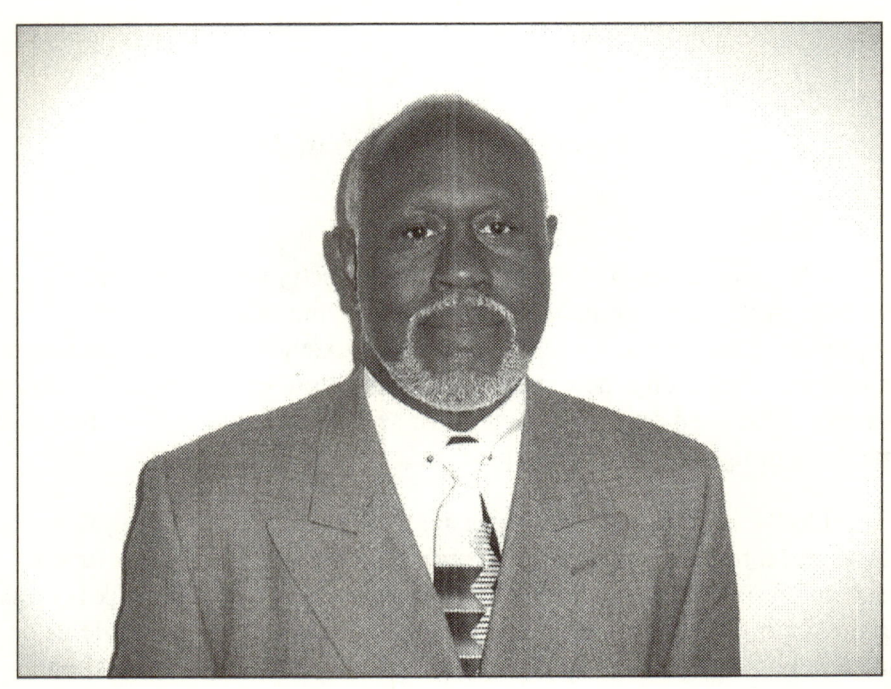

Reverend Isaac C. McCullough

Black Church Initiative of the Religious Coalition for Reproductive Choice - Washington, DC

B.S., Management and Human Resources, B.A., Psychology and Certificate, Religion and Bible Studies
In Ministry 20 years; Pastored Christ Community United Methodist Church for 7 years; Chair of the Board of Directors for Committed Caring Faith Communities (CCFC), Saint Louis, MO
Married (Glenda)

CRISIS IN THE BLACK CHURCH:

THE BLACK CHURCH

AND THE LIFE OF THE COMMUNITY

Reverend Isaac C. McCullough

Let us not forget the history of the Black Church as the cornerstone of the community for people of color. The church led the fight for the rights of our people, and not only people of color, but _all_ people. I have come to believe that the church has taken a back seat on many issues related to our spiritual, physical, mental and emotional health. To better understand our spirituality, we must deal with the issues that affect our thought process. It's of the utmost importance that we reach the spiritual soul of the people, which will in turn assist and encourage them to make right decisions before God, that they may be whole and complete in their existence.

Paul, in Galatians 5:16-26, gives useful information about the "flesh" which is comprised of our lusts, our passions, our 'humanness', and is the part of us that stands in opposition to God. As spiritual beings the evidence of Christ's life in ours includes love, joy, peace, patience, kindness, goodness, faithfulness, gentleness, and self-control. As *fleshly* beings, the evidence of the flesh includes immorality, impurity, sensuality, idolatry, sorcery, enmities, strife, jealousy, outbursts of anger, disputes, dissension in our relationships, envying, drunkenness, carousing, and things like these.

Tangibly, the flesh is not so much revealed in our human definition, but is ostensibly revealed in our most innate feature -- our spirituality -- which dictates our attitudes, desires, and lifestyles. Never think that just because you serve the Lord you won't be caught up in the trappings of the flesh. A person can serve God, make a wonderful public impression, and yet be struggling in the flesh.

The primary focus of the flesh is self-will, self-assertion, self-love, self-indulgence, self-pity, self-reliance, self-consciousness, self-righteousness, and self-glorification. However, to be successful in making correct, *Godly* choices, the central focus of the Spirit-filled life must always be Jesus Christ. As children of God, we have been given the power to say 'no' to our old way of living and thinking. Ask the Lord to reveal any evidences of the flesh in your life. Be willing to allow Him to strip away all that does not glorify Him.

It is apparent that in many areas of human life, the church is failing. The black church must begin to speak out about issues that affect and impact the total life of our people, not just members of the congregation but the community. Although this article is written to and for the black community, the information shared applies to people of all ethnic and racial groups.

As stated in I Corinthians 3:16 "Do you not know that you are the temple of God and that the Spirit of God dwells in you?" Knowing that you are a very special person to God and knowing that all people around the world are of utmost importance to God, we share hope that will encourage hearts to take care of God's temple. As spiritual leaders, it is important that we speak out about issues that impact our community. In our community, there are many issues that needs that we should be addressing on a daily basis: health issues; community relations; community development; community involvement; community violence; community employment; community jobs; community safe places for children, youth and senior adults for activities, and most of all, educating the community on all areas of live.

Listed below are some of the issues that affect the black church that spiritual leaders must become proactive and address regularly:

Family abuse – Let us remember that we are our brother's keeper, in Genesis 4:9, God asked Cain an important question: **"And the LORD said unto Cain, Where is Abel thy brother? And he said, I know not: Am I my brother's keeper?"** Jesus shares these words of importance to inform us that we are our brother's keeper in Matthew 25:34-40: **"Then the King will say to those on His right hand, 'Come, you blessed of My Father, inherit the kingdom prepared for you from the foundation of the** world: for I was hungry and you gave Me food; I was thirsty and you gave Me drink; I was a stranger and you took Me in; 'I was naked and you clothed Me; I was sick and you visited Me; I was in prison and you came to Me. "Then the righteous will answer Him, saying, 'Lord, when did we see You hungry and feed You, or thirsty and give You drink? 'When did we see You a stranger and take You in, or naked and clothe You? Or when did we see You sick, or in prison, and come to You?' "And the King will answer and say to them, 'Assuredly, I say to you, inasmuch as you did it to one of the least of these My brethren, you did it to Me."

Spouse abuse – we often turn our head the other way when we sense or detect that the relationship between a couple might be out of hand. Part of the problem is that we don't want to pry into others lives and it will appear that we are intruding in their affairs.

Parent abuse – more and more, we are hearing about parents and grandparents being abused by the ones they love. Although the Church of God (not the denomination), shares love, mercy, and grace with forgiveness, but yet we hurt the ones we love. Why is that? I am reminded that in the book of Proverbs chapter 22 we are to *train* our children; too many children are growing up without training and love. We are reminded that, "Foolishness is bound in the heart of a child; but the ***rod of correction*** shall drive it far from him." Let's take a moment and reflect on ***rod of correction***, I believe that the ***rod of correction*** is the Word of God. If we are not properly training our children, then we can expect anything from them. I do believe that most of our children are deficient of love, and they are reaching out in anyway they can for help and love.

Child/children abuse – many of our children are being abused by parents and adults who should be providing care, love, support and most of all protection. What we may fail to understand is that most children who are abused, end up being abusers themselves. It may be that they are thinking this is the way life should be. We must provide protection and the church has to be involved in the life of family. The family is the oldest institution under heaven.

Sex abuse – We all know that substance abuse and sexual acts are just two of the culprits that wreak havoc in our world today. One of the major transmitters of HIV (human immunodeficiency virus) today is our sexual life style with multiple partners, which include MSM (**m**en having **s**ex with **m**en), IV (intravenous) Drug users, men with both male and female partners, some males admitting that they enjoy sex with both genders of the human species, referred to as bi-sexual and/or gay, while some other men have sex with both genders of the human species, but deny they have sex with men, or that they are gay or bi-sexual, referred to as DL (Men on the Down Low). What is a sad commentary of our society today is, HIV is 100% preventable, but for many of us we prefer the 30 seconds' thrill of pleasure that alters the remainder of life forever. Part of the sadness in our country today, is that blacks make up only 12 to 13% of the population, but in every age category we have the highest percentage of HIV/AIDS victims.

It is important that the spiritual community begin dialogue. Healing and understanding develops our faith journey. In the black church, we are slow to speak out and function with a closed mind when it comes to talking about sex, sexuality and all issues pertaining to relationships. Relationships are essential to every individual. We look to various vices to establish relationships and many of these vices are not healthy for us.

How is it possible to prevent HIV/AIDS? The _only_ fool-proof, 100 percent effective-rated, way to prevent infection by this dread disease (or any other STD, for that matter) is to abstain from sexual activity until united in Holy Matrimony, with both partners abstaining until marriage. There are various safeguards that God has provided to ensure our protection. Today, it is important that both individuals establish and maintain a monogamous relationship. This is _central_ towards the prevention of contracting HIV/AIDS in sex, while also not getting involved with intravenous drug usage and sharing needles.

The question today is 'why is the church (the black church) not making their number one priority the addressing of issues that is currently destroying the life of our community and world?' As stated in Ecclesiastes 3:7b "A time to keep silent, and **a time to speak**." It is now time that we as spiritual leaders establish dialogue and address the issues in our congregations that they may not only grow spiritually, but physically.

Let us not forget that our body is the temple of God and we must begin to treat it as such. It should be our goal to minister to the *whole* person. We must address issues that are people-destroying and we must not label others based on what we feel or think; this is not godly. As Spiritual Leaders, we must never forget that it is the Word of God that transforms and changes the heart of mankind as addressed to the Romans in Romans 12:2. We are the messengers of God -- to share information to assist the people in making good and sound decisions each day of their life.

In our society today, the world is filled with all types of messages and most of them are not healthy, nor are they Godly. It is important we internalize these messages with a focus on what God has said from His Holy Written Word. Let us take time to meditate on God's Word while fasting and praying. The strength of our lives is in our power to pray, that we can face the challenges that come our way. With the Word of God and prayer, lives will be forever changed...

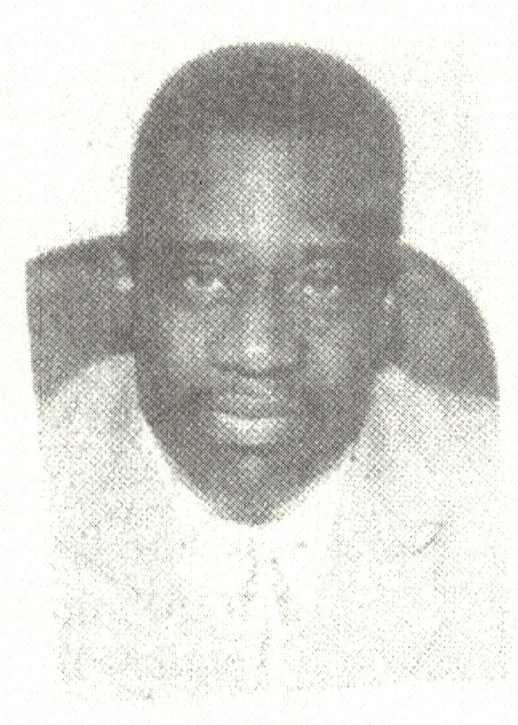

Elder Andrew J. Latchison, Jr.

Pastor of WellSpring International Ministries, Inc.
B.A. Education, St. Louis Public School Teacher for 28 years;
Originator of "BodyBuilders"© and "Gathering of Eagles"© Men's and
Women's Conferences; in Ministry over 30 years, Pastor for 27 years
Married (Hope)

"Eric's Confession"

Elder Andrew J. Latchison, Jr.

There's an old saying 'what you don't know can't hurt you' but that is a spurious and incorrect statement. Most of what we don't know we simply lay aside, ignore or develop an antipathy towards, until either directly or inadvertently we are affected. If there is an indictment against the church and its people, it lies in our ignorance of the facts and our ability to ignore the facts that causes much harm.

For years we have watched our loved ones die and have whispered our trepidation to one another. We have pointed our fingers and have even walked on the other side, in another aisle to avoid contact with folks who may appear to be 'sick.' We didn't even have a name for it many years ago, but we knew something was *wrong*, something was *different*. Our attitude has been if we ignore some things it will eventually go away – but not THIS... We had a chance to deal with it, to educate and postulate – but our posture was that of secrecy and desertion. We just let folks *DIE...*

We, the people of God, possess the greatest keys of reconciliation, hope and *life*. Supposedly, we have love and compassion. Jesus said that the world would know us by our love. The shame of it all is our continued turning away -- apostasy, if you will. The greatest way to control a crisis is to confront it head on. But no, we are *yet* turning away.

Because of our lack of *compassion*, many of our family, friends and church brethren have died, I believe, before their time. However, there is still time for us that remain to inform our people about the consequence of ignorance towards this horrific disease: AIDS. We must educate our children, our youth about the effects of AIDS and how they can make a *difference* in the world by not becoming a statistic. Then, we must bring our head out of the clouds and humble ourselves to extend a hand, a heart of relief and healing to the sick and wounded. God holds us responsible!

I want to tell you a story of my once-detestable attitude towards AIDS and one of its unfortunate victims – but how God brought victory into a crisis situation. It became a 'Christ-*is*' approbation.

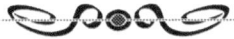

On Independence Day, July 4, 1993, one of my members claimed his freedom and gained a new lease on life. Eric was a tall, stately, well-dressed though rather obese, sophisticated young man. He was always well-groomed, poised and 'grand'. Generally, I am drawn to those kinds of folks but for some reason, I dared not get close to Eric. He had always been very cordial and respectful to me and just *adored* Dorcas, hailing her 'Ms. Wonderful First Lady.'

Eric was homosexual and *definitely* 'out of the closet', not concerned with what others thought of him. It wasn't that he necessarily flaunted it; he just seemed to 'wear' his homosexuality like a garment. Whenever he was around, Eric attracted many of like kind. They would flock to him because he had great character. But I was not only distant but totally biased against Eric and 'his kind'.

I remember how they used to come into our sanctified church when I was a teen and just stand in the hallway and kiss on each other and hug, rubbing all over each other. I said there were just *too many women*, all *kinds* of women – even those who look like men. There was just no reason for a man to want another hard man. God had made Adam for Eve, not Adam for Albert, Eve for Eva. That always went over good with church folk but the 'homos' slashed my tires and sometimes even knocked out the windows in my car. I even received threatening phone calls after many of my sermons. So, Lord, you know I didn't want any of those 'things' in my church...

I'm not so sure if it was good or bad but I began to think of the families of these 'wayward' folk – that they needed support, teaching and mentoring even if I wasn't comfortable with their shady kin. I began to have a hunger for a ministry towards these families and several families joined almost at once, loving our church and its music. However, Eric's family never joined. Eric one day called to ask if his sister, Pat, could have her wedding ceremony at our beautiful church and I immediately said yes. I had met Pat a few years back and was obliged to perform the ceremony myself. At the wedding, I began to notice Eric's weight loss. He explained that since he was a professional chef he had gotten sick of food, and was becoming a vegetarian. Even though he also claimed to have been on a diet, Eric seemed to have lost the weight so quickly.

After a while, church members began to ask questions. Eric's clothes were literally falling off of him. He didn't look healthy. His skin began to take on an ashy, grayish look. He suddenly became withdrawn and distant but attempted to act cheerful. When the Spirit was high and the saints would go into praise, Eric would shout and cry louder and longer than anyone else.

Afterwards, he would cough and sweat profusely so much that he would have to be taken out of the sanctuary. We all began to suspect the worst. Eric called and asked for prayer, stating that he was very ill but never disclosed the nature of his condition. He wanted to come before the church with a statement, if possible. He said he wanted to 'bare his soul.' The Sunday Eric requested was to be the 4th of July, Independence Day.

We had early service that particular Sunday due to the parade in the downtown area where the church was located. After a certain time, all of the streets would be blocked off and there would be no way in or out. Our deacons began devotion with very few present. However, they all seemed to come at once – Eric being in the number with several of his family members. His mother, sister, aunts, uncles and others took up the first three pews. I went through the first portion of the service and then stated that Eric had something to share with the church. Lord, you *know* how I felt. I was afraid at first but felt somehow that you, Lord, would get the glory out of all of this!

Eric confessed that he had AIDS and his time wasn't long, but that he had given his life to Christ and was filled with the Holy Spirit. He said he regretted his past undisciplined, rambunctious lifestyle but when you're young you sometimes feel invincible, like nothing can hurt you. Eric stated that he had been hard-headed and disobedient. He had a good family that loved him and a pastor who preached the Word but somehow he had turned it all away – until now. He cried and exclaimed that he wasn't sad because he was dying; they were only tears of joy. He was praising God because he was finally living. He told the other fellows who had adopted his past lifestyle that it was *wrong*. And no matter what anybody said to condone it, it was *wrong* and God didn't like it, but if they came to the Lord He would forgive.

Eric stated that he now had something that the world didn't give and certainly couldn't take from him – life, peace and salvation. He extended his arms to his family who came to embrace and rejoice with him. And Lord did we *shout*! There was more joy in that place that day than the fireworks going off outside! I preached from the subject "Free At Last" (I Corinthians 5:17). Seven souls gave their lives to the Lord that Sunday. A few weeks after that special Sunday, Eric died.

Lord, thank you for Eric's independence – and *mine*. I could never thank you enough for teaching me that *all souls* are yours…

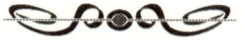

CHOICE and CONSEQUENCE

It's All About _Choice_...

The chapters of this book reveal some of the most serious flaws in our human character. Each of the 'deficiencies', a/k/a 'addictions', discussed have led to tragedy: lost family relationships, lost friendships, lost self-esteem, lost reputations, lost innocence, lost jobs, lost trust, lost health, lost futures, lost dreams, lost lives – lost _souls_. What will it profit a man if he should gain the whole world – and lose the _only_ thing he was given responsibility for -- _himself_?

Our _appetites_, our _cravings_, our _hunger_, our _greed_ have gotten us into deep trouble. And the sad reality is that each time we give in to our various lusts, we come up feeling more and more empty, guilty and unfulfilled. Pastor Charles Roach, one of St. Louis' most renowned pastors, accurately stated: "There is a crisis in communicable disease in our community... because there is a crisis in human behavior. We cannot expect to win any battle with disease unless there be a _change in human behavior_." Also clearly, there can be no change in human behavior unless there is a change in human _will_...

The great controversy between good and evil has not been waged on some far distant battleground but rather 'up close and personal' in the recesses of the human mind. It is the human will, with its powerful liberty to choose, which determines the course of each individual's life – based on five senses. If everyone could appreciate the import and magnitude of personal choice and the ramifications of making wrong choices, _millions_ of lives would be kept from destruction. The choices we make, _make us_...

The late Flip Wilson during his variety show would sometimes portray Geraldine, a loose-lipped, sarcastic woman. Geraldine made this statement famous: "The _devil_ made me do it!" Yes, the devil _is_ responsible for an awful lot: _"And the Lord said unto Satan, "From where are you coming?" And Satan answered the Lord and said, 'From going to and fro in the earth and from walking up and down in it'_ (Job 2:1). 1 Peter 5:8 gives us the _reason_ for Satan's pacing in the earth: _"Be serious, watchful; because your enemy the devil, as a raging lion, walks about, seeking out whom he can destroy."_

More times than we would probably care to admit, however, the devil had little if anything at all to do with many of our choices. Realistically, we just *wanted* to... In the case of Eve, she barely heard a word the devil said to her. The tree was pretty and the fruit was pleasant to the eye. The fact of the matter is that we put up very little struggle against temptation. Anything that appeals to our senses -- sight, taste and *P-LEASE* don't let it *feel* good, here we go – *AGAIN!!!* This present era is perhaps the most addicted *ever* to have lived on the face of the planet! We form addictions to everything: sex, drinking, smoking, drugging, gambling, eating – and the list goes on...

Throughout history, as well as the Bible, the same dynamic has been in operation. Satan has *without fail* employed the use of the five senses in causing humans to err. He has no other access to the mind than through our gifts of sight, hearing, touch, smell and taste. Since God created the mind to instinctively submit to whatever enters through these means, this is where the devil directs his strongest attacks. Satan himself cannot *force* entry through the senses. Therefore, he utilizes his most prevailing influences by means of our touch, sight, etc. in an effort to gain entry into the mind. He barrages the senses with seductive illusions, until we *give him* access to our mind and thoughts.

It is called *temptation*. Satan has used his cunning devices of sensory overload for thousands of years, is well experienced -- and it has *always* worked. Because the devil knows that humans are sensual creatures (it is how we acclimate to our world) and basically egocentric in nature, he doesn't have to employ any other technique than attractive illusions. It worked back in the Garden – and it *still* works.

In the error of miscalculating our strengths and weaknesses, we play a *dangerous* game of Russian Roulette with Satan, destroying our defenses by *lingering* in the atmosphere of temptation. It is this very lingering, hesitation, or second glance which Satan uses and embellishes to *blossom* in our thought processes. Here lies the very origin of every human indiscretion ever perpetrated: the intrinsic predilection to gratify the senses. How often has a full-blown act of sin resulted from just *a look*? Satan gets busy with his sensory illusions, making things look *a lot* better than they actually are and *here we go!*

We always quote James 4:7b: "***Resist*** *the devil and he will flee from you.*" However, we make a *huge* boo-boo for not giving *more* notice to James 4:7a: "***Submit*** *yourselves therefore to* <u>*God*</u>." Regrettably, we all know the result of paying more attention to 4:7(b) than 4:7(a): "Satan, now *gone… Go* on… Git ye *behind* me… (Pause) What-what-what you dur'n?… Aw *naw*, Satan, I didn't mean like *that*!!" In the future, let us make it a practice to submit to God *first,* to receive the power we need to resist the devil.

In a sermon to literally thousands some years ago the dynamic pastor and evangelist, Bishop Noel Jones, made an impassioned plea that has remained with me to this day: "*Stop* doing permanent kinds of things in temporary situations. For what it takes 15 minutes to do can take you *15 years* to get out of." The concept is powerful: JUST STOP… STOP the behaviors that are harmful. STOP hanging with people who negatively influence you. STOP making unwise and unsafe choices. God has given us a mind to *think* with, to *choose* with and to *refuse* with. We must learn to employ the power of a '*positively* NO.' If a certain place or person presents a particular enticement which is hard to resist, we have the *power* and *responsibility* of slamming the door closed on temptation. God will not do for us what He has given *us* the power and ability to do ourselves.

God is not going to *force us* into obeying His word but desires obedience produced from a heart of love for Him. Someone who creates a robot programs it to do exactly what he wants it to do. God did not create human beings as robots. That would be the same as saying that we have no choice. God did not make us in such a way that our obedience to Him would be automatic. He granted us *free will*, so that we could obey because we *love* Him.

In your personal relationships, what means more to you: when someone does something for you because he is *forced* to do it or because he *wants* to? In our human relationships do we want *forced* love, or *forced* devotion? Do we feel good when our spouse or otherwise never acknowledges us to friends? Do we want to continually follow up behind someone to make sure they do the right thing? Do we want to continually have to change ourselves in order to keep someone attracted to us? The answer is a resounding NO…

Well, God doesn't want it either. All He wants is for man to *acknowledge* Him. The word 'acknowledge' means to admit, to confess, to recognize, to allow, to accept, to concede, to comply – and to 'let in'. He desires for us to get to know Him willingly, trust and serve Him continually -- because we *love* Him. And when it's all said and done, this is the *only* thing that will keep us from doing wrong – thinking about how much we love God and don't want to hurt Him when we act contrary to His word.

It's not much to ask of us because here's the key: God loved us so much that He created us in His image, after His likeness. He brilliantly, thoughtfully and compassionately modified Earth into a paradise for man's habitation. After Adam and Eve's disobedience, it ripped God's heart out, since they now had to die. He couldn't go back on His word because He's a holy God who doesn't lie. He watches over His word to perform it and whatsoever He has said will come to pass. So we can *choose* to love God. And that love—not our earlier life, not our acquired faults, not our inherited tendency to do wrong—is the key to our future. Such love is what each of us needs in order to survive and pass Life's test.

All He wants of us is to come to Him as a child, knowing nothing. The Kingdom belongs to the 'child', who doesn't have to struggle to achieve any state of spiritual loftiness or intellectual understanding. Not hung up on degrees or accomplishments, not boasting of spiritual perfectionism and achievements, not hemming and hawing to get into good standing. Just *come* and take advantage of the marvel of God's grace.

Does this mean that genes, environment, personal experience are irrelevant? *No.* God *recognizes* each of these as important influences. Everyone born on the face of the earth is a composite of four primary elements: environment (which includes upbringing), personal character-istics, life experiences and choices. These dynamics are tossed in tandem, merging to create whoever we become. For example, my St. Louis environs and upbringing, my personality, life experiences and choices have bred in me a rather bizarre amalgamation of a reserved, non-effusive, astute, spiritual, direct, tenacious, intuitive, voracious reader, practiced listener and open-minded introvert. As a result, I was labeled 'different' – even as a child. But we are *all* different – because no one of us has experienced all of the exact, identical primary elements.

Parental training, environment and negative experiences can have a tremendous impact on a child -- for good or for bad. Today, these dynamics are all evident in our lives. For example, some of us face challenges right now as a result of being 'different' and having difficult childhoods. These *sore* points are as much an intricate part of our lives as the *good* points. We are a composite or finished product of all that we have experienced. Many continue in the pattern of abuse because that, too, has become a bad habit we have become accustomed to. But we can take comfort from the Bible that we are *not* doomed to repeat the same mistakes over and over. There is no reason we have to perpetuate the sins of the past *or* the present – whether the mistakes are ours, our parents', our grandparents' -- *whoever*.

We *all* have obstacles to overcome—perhaps a lifetime of bad habits and harmful influences that distort our thinking. But we may take comfort in the certainty that God knows, see and cares. He is aware of the negative influences we struggle with -- whether inherited or acquired. He understands how these have affected us (Ephesians 4:22-24). But God's spirit can produce beautiful, precious qualities in all of us. The first of these is love. God wants us to *choose* to love even our enemies, and those that have done us great harm. He wants us to choose to abundantly *live* – and the only way we can do this is by faith in God and His Word.

You read earlier the *horrific* experience of Evangelist Ruth Nichols, my sister, who was brutally gang-raped when she was 15 years old. She has often related the story of how one night while conducting revival at a local church, one of the teen boys (now a man) that had raped her walked into the church. She recognized him immediately and said her heart skipped several beats. He proceeded to walk towards the pulpit, Bible in hand, 'happy in Jesus.' Ruth stated that she could do little else than just sit with her mouth gaped open in *shock* as he proceeded to go from one end of the pulpit to the other greeting other ministers. She stated that before he reached her, she suddenly became nauseous and ran outside. Not stopping until she had reached the corner, Ruth clung to a light post, sobbing. "How *could you*? How *could you* forgive this man who *beat* me, *raped* me and left me for *dead*?, she screamed at God. *"He should be <u>dead</u> by now for what he did to my life!"*

Ruth honestly thought she had gotten past that experience and was unaware of the anger, bitterness and hatred she yet retained. Suddenly, a subtle breeze came from *nowhere* and a gentle voice within her said: "I forgave him because he *asked* me to. Didn't I show <u>you</u> mercy and forgive <u>you</u> when you asked? " Ruth stated that she paused just long enough to ask forgiveness for not letting go of the bitterness and hatred of that past experience -- and ran so fast that she was back in the pulpit in 30 seconds flat. She ran with open arms to her past attacker, hugging and rocking him like an old friend.

The young man had come for service after hearing on the radio that "Sister Ruth" would be conducting the revival. It turns out that he had gotten saved at *another* service Ruth conducted, after hearing her testimony of deliverance from drugs. These are the words he said that night to her: "Sister Ruth, if it hadn't been for you and your testimony of deliverance, I would be dead *right now*. The Lord, *through you*, saved my life and now *I'm* in the ministry helping other drug addicts to Christ!" The young man never recognized her from that long ago, tragic time – and Ruth never told him…

God wants us to *choose* forgiveness. The Apostle Paul, who volunteered himself as a *coat rack* at the stoning of Stephen, knows more than *anyone* about the necessity to 'forget things in the past' and wrote, *"I do not count myself to have attained or arrived. But this one thing I must do* (the present)*: forget those things which are behind me* (the past)*, and reach for those things which are before me* (the future)*. I strive, I push, I press towards the attainment of a greater calling of God in Christ Jesus"* (Philippians 3:13, 14).

In order for each of us to move forward into our destiny, we *must* let go of the past. Keep the past *in the past*! Don't keep dredging it up. It's a ploy of the enemy to keep us bound, hopeless and helpless. Dr. Wayne Dyers once said: "Give up your personal history. If you don't have a history, you don't have to live up to it. Pick up your past and embrace it, then toss it away – and march into the *now*."

Satan's ultimate goal is to steal the *God-breathed* purpose that each of us was placed on earth to fulfill. He knows that if he can get to us through our various lusts and appetites, these can be used to *take us out*.

He can stop our purpose, by stopping *us*. But each of us was created by Jehovah God for a purpose, *with* purpose. When we realize this, we can say like Kevin A. Williams, a truly gifted painter: "I'm not an artist. I'm only the *brush* He uses." Make it a point as Dr. Dwayne Dyer once said: "Don't die with your music still in you." Bless the world by letting it know what your *'song'* is – you are the *only one* that can 'sing' your song.

I am especially inspired when I see people who have a handicap but are not 'handicapped'. We can each possess as many disabilities as is allowed and yet not be disabled. One of the groups that inspire me tremendously is the *'Foot and Mouth Artists'* of Atlanta, Georgia. Most of these *incredible* artists are paraplegics, or were born without arms but use their feet or mouth to produce art that would make Monet's work look amateurish. By using their God-given talent they are self-sufficient.

None of us were born perfect, without flaw; we each have our own set of deficiencies – whether innate, inherited or acquired. Don't ever think that you were singled out by Life to be picked on. We've *all* experienced terrible times. But there is one thing that makes all the difference in the world and as long as we possess it, any *beautiful*, positive thing is possible: we have the *breath of God*. As long as we have that breath, whatever we haven't accomplished for whatever reason – we yet have another chance. Let us make use of *every* breath, *every* chance we have, to utilize the gift or talent He gave us – and therefore fulfill our purpose. God wants us to choose to live life to the fullest -- *not recklessly*. Remember, true 'living' does not mean doing things that end up killing us.

God wants only the very best for us, His children. He knows we are fallible and incapable of changing ourselves. That is why the Holy Ghost was sent, not to *make* us live right -- He is *not* the Enforcer -- but help us to make right choices. Again, we must *choose* to let the Holy Ghost do his job in us, which is to lead and guide us into all truth. The spirit of God can help us make broad changes in ourselves. He can turn a *mess of a life* into a *miracle*. That's what change is – *a miracle*, and personal change never happens without God. In the words of Evangelist Ruth Nichols: "But if *you* make the *choice, He'll* make the *change!*"

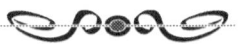

"The Truth Shall *Make* You Free"

What is it about the truth that sends us reeling, grappling for something to shore us up? Even though we may *think* the truth, or *hear* the truth, it is next to impossible for us to *speak* or *admit* the truth. Is it that we *prefer* lies and fairy tales to the truth, or is it because we've been faking it for so long we really don't know what the truth is? Brennan Manning once said, "The dichotomy between what we say and what we do is so pervasive in church and society that we actually come to believe our illusions and rationalizations, clutching them to our hearts like favorite teddy bears."

Imposters at heart always prefer *appearances* to *reality*. When they look in the mirror not liking what they see, cosmetics, makeup, padding in essential places, are used to create an acceptable image. We 'wear masks', 'put on a good face,' 'keep up appearances', 'save face' – and any number of other glib modifications to disguise our true self. We do quite a bit with our face -- except 'face' facts. Self-deception prevents us from realizing the truth of who we *really* are, which ultimately prevents us from getting the help we *desperately* need to be true to ourselves and everyone else.

Many have been guilty of feigning and pretension because of *fear*—fear of not being accepted, fear of abandonment, fear of what people will say or think, fear of the consequence of being honest or true. Fear binds, paralyzes and prevents one from moving forward. The Bible suitably equates 'fear' to 'torment'. It is *tortuous* to pretend to be something or someone you are not. When we attempt to be something other than what we were *created* to be, it is impossible to be good at it.

I John 4:18 says, *"There is no fear in love; but perfect love cast out all fear…He that fears is not made perfect love."* Freedom in Christ produces a healthy disregard of peer pressure, people-pleasing and public opinion. It is impossible to be *true* and *truthful* if we adapt to the controlling pressure of people-pleasing. Attitudes will vacillate spastically, based on the group, environment and circumstances. Thus, we become frauds, hypocrites. Did you know that the word 'hypocrite' actually means 'poor actor'? You can never walk in freedom or deliverance attempting to please people.

While the question 'why would anyone *want* to please people?' is poised in air, it needs to be pointed out that a great many lives have been ruined by taking this route. Dark deeds have long been committed by those too weak to say 'no' to peer pressure because their desire to fit in or be liked wins out over morality and common sense. Some people simply cannot bypass attempting to gain the notice or favor of other people – doing whatever it takes to win that 'friendship'. However, friendship that is garnered at the sacrifice of *self* is never worth it. Friendship that is 'bought' or gained through deception will not last. Those who truly love you will love you no matter what. You don't have to put on airs, or step out of your normal character – they will simply love you because you are uniquely *you*. Be true to yourself – and we each have our own truth...

Your truth and *my* truth will always be different because as individuals, we are different. As stated earlier, four basic fundamentals mold us, *shape* us into whoever we become: environment (upbringing), personal qualities, life experiences – and choices... Many might scramble to say that 'genes' play a heavy-duty part in who we are. I'll go along with that theory to an extent; *however*, genes actually play an *optional* part in our maturation, unique and final development. (She's *crazy!* Genes are a pattern that is stamped on the *unique* structure of our entire composition. They are unchanged!)

Do you know what the word 'unique' means? It means: single, sole, only, exclusive, one of a kind... Genes can determine what *family* you're in. Genes can determine your eye, hair and skin color – but *not* your destiny. There are no two people on the face of the earth with the exact same genetic pattern or DNA – not even the dead ancestors we want to pin the blame on for our messed up reality.

Sorry to bust your bubble but we have used the crutch of 'generational curses' far too long, far too much. And we do it to provide what we deem is a reasonable excuse for the failure of our *choices*. In this way we can better live with the consequences -- distancing ourselves from the potent equation of personal choice, result, blame and the ensuing guilt that is always associated with blame. *No one* wants to be blamed for ruination or failure – personal or otherwise.

It is much easier to develop the deception that because of the dead ancestors we are the way we are. It is almost *comforting* when we believe 'I can't help it. I *have* to do it. It's in my genes'. *Or,* 'you know, I have these *bad genes* from both my Mama *and* my daddy's side... *Or,* '*I* was abused so that's why I'm an abuser'. How long are we going to hold on to excuses and not face the truth, which is we are the way we are by *choice*?

How else do you explain a young man or woman raised in the projects, who saw violence of all type, was exposed to drugs, gangs and everything else that accompanies abject poverty. Yet, they became a doctor. Despite the fact their mother, father, uncle, auntie, grandmother, grandfather, sisters, brothers, etc. were alcoholics, abusers, sexual predators and the whole gamut of what is worst in families, they became a doctor. Though they were found in a *trashcan* at birth, were sexually and physically abused throughout childhood, they became a doctor. Though they were timid, introverted and not particularly good in school, they became a doctor.

In this scenario we can rule out genes, environment, upbringing, and personality traits. The only factor that we can adhere to is *choice*. He or she *chose* to overcome all other obstacles to become a doctor. This works also in the reverse: a child is born into a rich, powerful and prominent family but is now a bum living on the street. *Choices...*

"And you shall know the truth, and the truth shall make you free" (John 8:32). It is only 'the truth' that will free us. God's Word is truth – and it can *cut you up...* Many people prefer to use 'set you free', which to me evokes the mental impression of a lovely woman, running in slow-motion through a field of meadow flowers, smiling as she releases white doves into a pristine blue sky -- a *gentle* release without effort, without pain. A soft breeze is blowing all around, rustling up the soothing sounds of nature. Maybe there's a brook or pond close by, with glistening-gorgeous white swans floating ever so gently across the rippled water... Can you picture it?

Okay, now *snap out of it* because 'the truth' *I'm* referring to *HURTS*! It is *not* gentle! Renowned St. Louis pastor, Bishop Michael West, preached something recently that has remained with me: "Many of us are locked up in our past, and some are so caught up in the present that they don't have a future. Though the effects of condemnation are real, God is not interested in condemning you. God has forgiven us sometimes of some of the worse mess we have done, but we don't have the wherewithal to forgive *ourselves*"… And *that* is the key to ending a great deal of physical, emotional and spiritual abuse to *ourselves*!

A number of us are self-injurious in that we have internalized negative things that have turned *toxic*. Just as surely as if we take a knife and carve into our own flesh, we are self-injurers. Many have become so bitter until physical, chronic conditions have developed: high blood pressure, diabetes, heart trouble, mental angst, strokes, and even *cancer*. That *rape*, that bitter *divorce*, that *abandonment*, that *abuse*, that family *misunderstanding*, that *lie* told about you, or that *you* told – *let it GO!!!* Whatever happened in the past can't be fixed and *accept* that. But choose to be present, *in* the present. Decide to do what is right *today*…

Many others have taken on dangerous, unhealthy habits and are, in essence, committing *suicide*. Suicide is not only being committed by someone who takes a gun and blows their head off. Many of us are committing suicide *slowly* by justifying our negative behaviors, placating bad habits and giving in to even the *tiniest* trace of temptation. Whether you use a gun, or utilize the slow, tortuous method of bad habits and risky behaviors the end result will be the same: death by your own hand.

I can well relate to the *wrenching, tugging, pulling, yanking, twisting* that is involved in '*making*' one free. It has to be that way because we become so attached to long-held habits and long-standing patterns of abusive behaviors, though they are *wrong,* harmful to our physical and spiritual well-being, and against God's word. Oftentimes we act as if we are impervious to consequences because of our title, our position, our money, our family name, our education, 'cause we *bad*… **The same choices produce the same set of consequences**!

Truth requires honesty and courage to admit our addictions and hang-ups. In AA, you must first admit you are an alcoholic to stay in the program. The logic is that if you cannot openly admit you have a problem it is impossible to be helped. *"He that covers his sins shall not prosper"* (Proverbs 28:13a). The person will continue in the same pattern of abusive alcoholism simply because they cannot accept the truth of who they are.

Honesty involves a surrendering of will to face the truth of who we are, regardless of how unpleasant this proves to be. *"But whoever confesses and forsakes his sin shall receive mercy"* (Proverbs 28:13b).

Paul said in Hebrews 12:1b, 2: *'Let us lay aside every weight and the sin that does so easily hinder us, and let us run with determination the race that is set before us. Looking unto Jesus'...* We can't hold on to negative things in our past and succeed; neither can we run the race of Life with encumbrances. In this verse it's as if Paul is saying: *'Now, I realize you can't just <u>throw</u> this particular habit or addiction down because you apparently like doing it. But if you want to stay in the race, not having to be called out because you smoke and can't catch your breath, make an effort and choose to <u>put</u> it aside.'* We *must* stay in the race, running with determination – *always* looking unto Jesus to strengthen us so that we may be able to complete our course, fulfill our purpose.

Paul also says to 'put aside *the* sin'. Personally, I don't think Paul meant sin in general, but rather a *specific* one. There is always that *one thing* we love above anything else: sex, smoking, gambling, drinking, drugs, eating too much, gossiping, etc. And we *know* it's wrong but we just *gotta* have it! (Or *do* it...) It's like the time I saw a man smoking a cigar while hooked up to an *oxygen tank*. Or like the woman running Flo Valley's track – while eating the biggest bag of the greasiest chips *they make*! We all have *somethin'* that we simply can't resist, <u>*can't*</u> seem to let go – even though it may be the very death of us...

I don't know what yours is and you don't know what mine is but the *truth is* we all have *something* making us trip. Paul said to 'lay aside' every weight and *the* sin that <u>*so easily*</u> besets you. Meaning, whatever you like may hold no enticement for *me* and I can refuse it with no problem. *You* may smoothly pass the test for something that holds a great deal of attraction for me. There are definitely things we can say 'no' to quite effortlessly. *BUT* there is always that *one thing* that trips us up, that pops our top, butters our bread, turns us on, turns our head and just makes us *crazy*. We each know our individual indiscretion – that *specified* hang-up, that thorn in our flesh, that mote (or *2 x 4...*) in our eye. Many of our lives have been drastically altered because of that *specific* sin. It has cost us families, friendships, marriages, relationships, jobs, homes, property, cars, health, wealth, reputation -- *stripped us* -- but we keep goin' back...

But even more drastic than the loss of these things is the affect that it has on our relationship with God. God knows what we are, who we are, and *where* we are. We can't fool Him. God requires honesty: *'If we confess our sins He is faithful and just to forgive us, and to cleanse us from all unrighteousness. If we say we have no sin, we make Him a liar, and His truth is not in us'* (I John 1:9, 10). Getting honest with ourselves does not make us unacceptable to God. It draws us nearer and reinforces our relationship to Him.

When we accept responsibility for our choices and their consequences, when we accept ownership of our powerlessness and acknowledge our helplessness, then God's grace brings renewal and acceptance. We don't have to fall out and *beg* His forgiveness. We don't have to go into detail about our sorrow -- just *show up* in prayer; spend some time with the Father. Talk to Him like you would a good friend – no airs, no special words – just tell Him what you feel. Yes, He already knows but sometimes He just likes to hear your voice…

The miracle is that God loves us *in spite of* us. Romans 8:31b, 32, 35 (paraphrased*): "If God be for us, who can be against us? He that did not spare His own son but gave him as a sacrifice for us all, will surely not withhold anything from us…Who shall separate us from the love of Christ? Shall misfortune, suffering, abuse, deprivation, helplessness, danger or weapon? No, in all things we are more than conquerors because He loves us. Therefore, I am convinced that neither death, nor life, angels nor governments, no authority, nothing in the past, present, nor future, height, depth, nor any other being shall be able to disconnect us from the love of God, which is in Christ Jesus"…*

For this reason, life is worth living. God *accepts* us and He won't stop loving us even though we become discouraged and our grip on Him may give way. The power in this is that *He's* holding onto *us* and won't *ever* let go. And when we realize that God accepts us, there is no need to wear masks any longer. There is no need to give in to peer pressure or people-pleasing; and it doesn't matter who may reject us. We are loved and accepted by *The Best*…

"EVERYTHING IS VANITY"

Ecclesiastes begins with these words: *"The greatest vanity!'* the Preacher has said, *'the greatest vanity! Everything is vanity!' What profit does a man have in all his hard work at which he works hard under the sun?"* (Eccl. 1:2, 3) The Hebrew word for "vanity" literally means "breath." In his exclamation, you can sense Solomon's anguish at the reality of the fragility and futility of life. It indicates something that lacks firmness, stability and permanence. *"The greatest vanity"* well describes human affairs.

Next the Preacher mentions repetitious cycles in nature. Generations of people continually come and go, live and die, the sun keeps rising and setting, winds ever circle about and rivers constantly empty into the sea but never fill it (Eccl. 1:4-7). After reflecting on this, the wise king observed: *"All things are wearisome; no one is able to speak of it. The eye is not satisfied at seeing, neither is the ear filled from hearing. That which has come to be, that is what will come to be; and that which has been done, that is what will be done; and so there is nothing new under the sun."* —Eccl. 1:8, 9.

Solomon continues to ponder over the plight of all mankind in Ecclesiastes 2: *"I made me great works; I built me houses; I made me pools of water; I got me servants and maidens; I gathered me silver and gold. So I was great – then I looked on all the works that my hands had wrought and on the labor that I had accomplished. Behold, all was vanity and vexation of spirit. How does a wise man die? He dies the same as the fool. There is no remembrance of the wise more than of the fool forever"*...

The consideration of all these realities appeared to Solomon as "wearisome", or frustrating. It is, of course, true that the immensity and complexity of these cycles are such that a man could exhaust his entire life and never be able to comprehend the full sum of them. But keep in mind that Solomon is dealing with the same futility that we as imperfect humans face. For the one lacking divine insight, his temporariness and his inability to gain permanence produce a sense of futility and often cause him to search vainly for something different, something new—only to find that, in the final analysis, it is the same old story. This too brings no joy or satisfaction.

Case in point:

Just recently I attended a major awards ceremony, thanks to a *wonderful* friend who gifted me with two tickets to this event. (No, I am *not* going to tell which awards event it was...) And even though I was neither rich nor famous, there I sat rubbing elbows with true notables -- though I hadn't paid *one cent* to be in the same upfront seats they were. I hadn't made a movie or written a musical score but I was yet able to attend the same venue, eat from the same china, sit at the same table with those who had just won awards. And all the while I wondered: 'Is this *all* there is? No, there's just *gotta* be more'... With all the hoopla and fanfare that is always associated with an occasion of this caliber, after only a short while, it's over...

To tell you the truth, I would have been *sorely* disappointed had I done all that hard work that is involved in being 'recognized'. I would have felt like so many others who have struggled to get to a certain point in life or career only to discover: this is all there is... Paraphrased, Job said in Job 1:21: "*Naked* I came in and *naked* I'm going out" – and *nothing* we do between the two nakednesses will matter if we have not acknowledged God and obeyed His word in our living.

IF you have made this *world*, this *life*, this existence your sole raison d'être and have ignored the beckoning voice of God, your soul has no solace when the lights go out. There is no comfort for you when friends *walk out*, or health *gives out* -- or if the money and drinks *run out*. Then again, you may have *plenty* of money, with no danger of ever running out. Even then, money may buy you one of those 'sleep number' beds but not a good night's sleep. Money can purchase a state-of-the-art security *system* – but it can't buy you security. Money can buy the most expensive clock in the world – but it can't purchase you a *second's* worth of extra time...

"*What has it benefited you to have gained the whole world and lose your soul? What will you give Me in exchange for your soul?*" (St. Luke 12:16-21) was the question Almighty God posed to the 'rich man' in the

Bible who felt 'he *had it* like that.' He was going to tear down his barns, then build bigger barns, eat, drink, make merry and make plans – telling himself 'relax, man, you done *good*. You have enough stored up in the bank, stocks and bonds, real estate, investment accounts, mutual funds -- and the *Dow* rose today to a five-year high! You don't have a *thing* to worry about.' The rich man was gloating and chillin' when he heard the voice of God saying something that brought his one-man Oscars celebration to an end: "'*You fool. This night your soul is required of you. Then, whose shall those things be that you possess?' So is the man who is not rich towards God*"...

Please understand that God doesn't have anything against rich people -- to the contrary. It is only when we put these *'things'* -- money, social status, careers, fame, etc. -- ahead of the essentiality of knowing God that really makes Him unhappy. *"The Lord your God is a jealous God. You shall have no other gods before Me"* (Exodus 20:3-5). God is frustrated when anything other than establishing or strengthening our relationship with Him is placed in first priority. Priorities are important to God and He *must come first* in our lives. Keep in mind that He makes *us* His first priority -- *always* -- and wishes only to receive the same courtesy from His human creation.

Finally, Solomon -- after modulating over the transitory state of human existence, after perceiving that *'everything under the sun is vanity and vexation of spirit'* -- ultimately deduced: *"Let us hear the conclusion of the whole matter: Reverence God, and keep His commandments: for this is the sole responsibility of man. For He will bring every work into judgment, with every secret thing, whether it be good or whether it be evil."* (Ecclesiastes 12:13).

We are at our best when we make ourselves available to the Lord's will and are being used for His glory. Obedience to His Word can help us to avoid harm, and wasting time, effort and money trying to find fulfillment and happiness through sensual gratification. When this happens, we are fulfilling an important portion of the divine purpose for which we were designed and created.

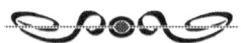

If nothing else you've read within these pages sinks in, the most crucial objective of this book is: *acknowledge God.* In all your ways -- rich ways, poor ways, right ways, wrong ways, happy ways, sad ways, up ways, down ways -- *acknowledge* Him. Be assured that God knows us so intimately, so *utterly* that He is acquainted with *all* our 'ways'. Stand fast in your trust that '*He knows the way that we take*' (Job 23:10) -- and when we have been tried, the Lord will bring us forth as gold...

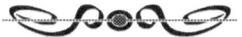